Introduction to Equine-Assisted Psychotherapy

A Comprehensive Overview

2nd Edition

Patti J. Mandrell, M.Ed., LPC
EAGALA-advanced

Copyright © 2014 by Patti J. Mandrell

Introduction to Equine Assisted Psychotherapy: A Comprehensive Overview

2nd Edition

By Patti J. Mandrell, M.Ed., LPC
EAGALA-advanced

Printed in the United States of America

ISBN

978-0-9916291-0-7

All rights reserved solely by the author. The author guarantees all contents are original and do not infringe upon the legal rights of any other person or work. No part of this book may be reproduced in any form without the permission of the author.

www.refugeservices.org

INTRODUCTION TO EQUINE-ASSISTED PSYCHOTHERAPY

Preface……………………………………………………………..v
    What is Equine-Assisted Psychotherapy Anyway?
    My Mission
    Acknowledgments

Part 1 – Foundation

Chapter 1 – Experiential Learning……………………………1
    Comparison to Traditional Therapy
    Various Methods to Experiential Learning
    Benefits of Processing

Chapter 2 – Key Theoretical Orientations ………………...14
    Cognitive-Behavioral Theory
    Reality Therapy
    Gestalt Therapy
    Brief Therapy
    Systems Theory

Chapter 3 – Why horses?..35
    Advantages of horses
    Comparison to other animals
    Horses as teachers

Chapter 4 – Benefits of Equine-Assisted Psychotherapy…….47
    Advantages to Equine-Assisted Psychotherapy
    Research
    Case studies
    Insights from other professionals
    Client testimonies

Part 2 – Treatment Team

Chapter 5 – The Role of the Mental Health Professional......76
    Tasks and skills needed
    Planning and facilitating individual sessions
    Planning and facilitating group sessions

Chapter 6 – The Role of the Horse Professional....................84
    Criteria for a safe EAP horse professional
    Tasks and skills needed
    Planning an individual session
    Planning group sessions

Chapter 7 – The Horse...94
    Horse psychology and body language
    Equine needs and attributes
    Horse cues
    Application to EAP

Part 3 – The Client

Chapter 8 – Who can benefit.....................................110
    Client structures
    Issues often addressed in EAP
    Common fears and misconceptions of clients
    Case summary

Chapter 9 – Working with specific age groups...............124
    Piaget's Cognitive Development Theory
    Erikson's Psychosocial Stages of Development
    How Age Impacts Equine-Assisted Psychotherapy

Chapter 10 – Working with groups............................135
    Benefits of group therapy
    Formation of the group
    Stages of group development

Part 4 – Safety

Chapter 11 – Physical and emotional safety..................153
    Physical safety
    Emotional safety

Chapter 12 – Setting up a session............................176
    Establishing a safe work area
    Tools and equipment used in facilitation
    Variety in equipment and therapy horses
    Guidelines in setting up an activity

Chapter 13 – Crisis Response...............................192
    Crisis intervention
    Action strategies for EAP professionals
    Legal implications
    Crisis Prevention

Part 5 – Multidimensional Processing

Chapter 14 – Components of processing....................204
    Four components of EAP processing
    Prioritizing and filtering observations
    Value of metaphors
    Why process?

Chapter 15 – Planning Sessions.............................223
    Incorporating client goals into the session
    Treatment planning
    Designing activities related to goals
    Choosing the appropriate horse and setting
    Filtering out personal agendas

Chapter 16 – Facilitating Sessions..........................233
    Treatment goal implementation
    Setting up the session
    How to conduct sessions
    Documenting Progress

Chapter 17 – Assessment and evaluation.....................247
    The importance of assessment
    Techniques and procedures
    Professional assessment and evaluation
    Program assessment – techniques and process
    Conclusion

Appendix..269

Sample Activities
    Group
    Family
    Individual

EAP Certification information

Code of Ethics

Bibliography..278

PREFACE

Being the first textbook written on the topic was an endeavor in itself. There is so much information, philosophy, and theory that come into play when you choose to include Equine-Assisted Psychotherapy into your toolbox of therapeutic tools. This endeavor has not been short-lived. I started this writing journey in 2002. Clients continue to take precedence as my writing time quickly slips away from me. In 2006, I published the first edition. Throughout the years, my understanding of EAP grows as clients and horses continue to take the session beyond where I had experienced it going before. So after fifteen years of facilitating the EAGALA model of EAP and hundreds of additional hours with clients, I am writing the second edition to this textbook. Personal growth in facilitation continues as I see the miracle of this work transform lives. The explanation and facilitation techniques of EAP continue to evolve through the years as experience helps us all become better facilitators; however, the core fundamentals of the approach remain the same. Fortunately, there is more research and information to scientifically support this work than available when the first edition was written. This field continues to grow exponentially.

I continue to be amazed at the power in this form of therapy when I step back and allow the process to take place before me without my orchestration. It is such a privilege to work with clients and walk with them through their most difficult moments. The horses aid in this process so beautifully – better than any intervention I could remedy in my office for sure!

My newest awareness is that the more I trust the process and get "myself" out of the way, the more room I leave for the client to find their own success and solutions. In this second edition, I have added the additional components and perspectives gained through the years in an attempt to give you an even more complete and thorough overview than before as I continue to peel away the layers upon layers of depth to this therapeutic approach.

What is EAP Anyway?

This question has been asked more times than I can keep track of. I have spent the past fourteen years trying to explain to others what Equine-Assisted Psychotherapy (EAP) is and what it is not. "I've got a horse that needs some therapy," they would laugh and say as they walked by. No, EAP is not psychotherapy for horses although I have seen some horses become more confident and expressive after being involved in several EAP sessions. The others would quickly interrupt as I attempted in my explanation of EAP saying, "Oh yeah, I have a friend whose daughter is doing that for her physical therapy." Again, the answer is no – EAP is not the same as hippotherapy or therapeutic riding. Nevertheless, I have seen many people with disabilities benefit from EAP. "Oh, so you teach the kids to ride. I know horses are good for teaching kids about responsibility and discipline." You are right; those are some benefits to horsemanship. However, EAP is not horsemanship nor is it about riding a horse at all!

So, you may be asking yourself now, "What exactly is Equine-Assisted Psychotherapy?" I'm so glad you asked. It will take the next seventeen chapters to explain to you what EAP truly is. By definition, EAP is a dawning approach to professional counseling that helps clients of all ages address behavioral, emotional, spiritual, and relational issues using horses as an intervention tool. EAP is a non-threatening and action-oriented team approach to counseling including a licensed counselor, horse professional, and horse(s). Equine-Assisted Psychotherapy helps clients cope with change and develop positive means of facing life's struggles through the use of activities and experiences with horses.

Many are still confused even after the definition is heard and the explanation has been made about what EAP is not. The best explanation for understanding it is to see it in action.

My Mission

So, knowing the amazing impact the horses are having for clients and fully understanding the complexity of Equine-Assisted Psychotherapy (EAP), I felt compelled to be an active participant in the promotion of EAP as it continues to gain support and credibility worldwide. My mission in writing *Introduction to Equine-Assisted Psychotherapy* is to:

- present you with a clear picture of how Equine-Assisted Psychotherapy can work as an interventional tool for clients
- provide you with a solid foundation of the theoretical and philosophical backbone of EAP
- assist you in distinguishing why horses over other animals
- dispel some of the misconceptions and myths about Equine-Assisted Psychotherapy, particularly the ones that confuse EAP with horsemanship, hippotherapy, and/or therapeutic riding
- aid in the respect for a balanced team consisting of horse professional, therapist, and horse
- offer information, not certification, about the versatile applications of Equine-Assisted Psychotherapy
- Contribute a quality introductory text to the EAP field

After reading this book, my goal is that you will hold a greater understanding and appreciation for the field of Equine-Assisted Psychotherapy. I feel confident that with the knowledge gained through reading this text combined with the experience gained through the Equine-Assisted Growth and Learning Association's certification program (EAGALA), you would hold a very complete understanding and ability to apply this therapeutic tool. Mastery is only achieved through practice – no book can give you that level of expertise.

My hope is that if you are interested in pursuing EAP as a component of your career that you will take the time to further your experience through certification and additional workshops. Equine-Assisted Psychotherapy is a very powerful tool. It is recommended that you only practice the activities presented in this text under the supervision of a certified EAP professional. Equine activities are highly active and participatory. Improper use of the activities described in this text may result in injury. I, the author, do not assume any liability for loss or damage, direct or consequential, to the readers or others resulting from the use of the materials contained in this textbook, whether such loss or damage results from errors, omissions, ambiguities, or inaccuracies in the materials contained herein or otherwise.

Having stated the disclaimer read forward and enjoy learning more about the dawning discipline of Equine-Assisted Psychotherapy. This won't be the last you hear of it.

Acknowledgements

Although only one author is listed on the cover of this book, I cannot take all the credit for this work. There have been so many key people involved in this process with me throughout the eleven years since this book was conceived. First and foremost, I have to thank my husband, and EAP horse professional partner, for his endless support and encouragement in sessions with clients as well as with the pursuit of this book. He always seems to know when to add pressure and/or release that pressure with clients and horses. This same quality was very helpful in keeping me focused on the book from time to time. Thanks for being such a great EAP horse professional, husband, and father. You are my inspiration! Thank you to my precious boys, Brady and Wyatt. You inspire me to be the best at all I do; not to mention, have given me so many opportunities to practice stepping back and trusting the process. You are my biggest fans. After all, EAP is a team approach, and this book was no exception. I could not have done this without MY team.

Also, a big thanks goes to Greg Kirsten and Lynn Thomas who sparked the passion within me by introducing me to EAP. I always knew horses had been therapeutic for me growing up but never knew what depth their presence could have for clients. Thanks for encouraging me to pursue EAP and allowing me to grow as EAGALA grows and this approach becomes better known. Thank you for all the opportunities to be in leadership in the organization and in the field of EAP. Your vision is changing the lives of so many!

Of course, this process couldn't have been done without help from editors and proofreaders. Thank you to my numerous intern students who put in many hours editing, researching, and helping me find the latest research to support this work. Your input and efforts were much appreciated. Also, a special thanks goes to Dr. Tootie Tatum who has put in endless hours to edit and consult with me about the textbook. Thanks for being there for me when I got bogged down and stuck. You always had a way of encouraging me to keep on going with this book. Your knowledge, experience, and love for animals have been invaluable in this process. You are a jewel!

Finally, I realize that an attempt to acknowledge everyone who has helped me along the way is impossible. I am indebted to so many clients, students, fellow trainers, trainees, horses, and individuals who have provided me with opportunities to craft and test many of these ideas. This book has made its way into the hands of professionals, educators, and horse lovers around the world. The feedback has been very positive and encouraging, thank you for your desire to learn about EAP and your amazing stories to support this approach. Thank you to my past, present, and future clients, for whom this book is written; you have provided me with multiple opportunities to learn, grow, and challenge myself professionally. Others have offered feedback and support, I am better for it.

About the Author:

Patti Mandrell, M.Ed., LPC, is cofounder of REFUGE Services, a non-profit organization in Lubbock, TX providing EAP services to individuals, groups, families, agencies, and businesses. Patti was the first licensed counselor in Texas to be nationally certified in EAP; and she and her husband, Randy, were the second team to be awarded advanced status in the world. She and her husband both are international trainers and approved mentors for the International Equine Assisted Growth and Learning Association. Patti received her Master's degree at Texas Tech University in Counseling Education and has been practicing EAP for the past fifteen years. She has been spotlighted and interviewed in numerous local, state, national, and international publications and television broadcasts promoting the use of EAP when working with clients. Patti has developed an EAP curriculum in conjunction with this textbook that is being taught at several universities and colleges around the world. She lives and practices in Lubbock, Texas with her husband Randy and two sons, Brady and Wyatt.

1 EXPERIENTIAL LEARNING

Objectives:
- **Define Experiential Therapy**
- **Explore various experiential approaches**
- **Discuss benefits of Experiential Therapy**

Experiential learning is learning by doing. It is the way humans learn best. As an ancient Chinese proverb eloquently and succinctly notes: "I hear and I forget. I see and I remember. I do and I understand." Today, biologists and neuropsychologists argue that humans are "hardwired" to learn this way. It has been estimated that while we remember only 20% of what we hear and 50% of what we see; we retain fully 80% of what we do. As a result, there is great momentum for understanding the nature and power of experiential education and how it can make use of the way the human nervous system is wired to learn (Smolowe, Butler, Murray, 1999). These activity-based experiences have greater sticking power than traditional-style training in which participants sit and receive information via lecture, overhead and video. Think about it – which do you remember better? The first time you cracked open a driver's manual – or the first time you turned the key in the ignition, shifted from park to drive and accelerated (Smolowe, Butler, Murray, 1999)?

Comparison to Traditional Therapy

The use of the outdoors, adventure, and wilderness for promoting personal and psychological development dates back to the earliest times. Myths and legends abound of young people embarking on adventurous journeys in order to complete a rite of passage into adulthood (Peel & Richards, 2005). As a result, it soon became evident that outdoor adventure could develop qualities such as hardiness, resilience, problem solving and the ability to work as a member of a team (Hopkins & Putnam, 1993). This realization led to the development of what is now known as outdoor-adventure therapy. **Outdoor-adventure therapy** is a type of therapy in which outdoor activities that are physically and/or psychologically demanding are used within a framework of safety and instruction to promote interpersonal and intrapersonal growth (Luckner

& Nadler, 1995). While the physical nature of the outdoor activities is often a part of experiential activities, physical fitness and physical skills are not the primary goals. The claim is that physical activities can be used as an effective medium for participants to recognize and understand their own strengths, weaknesses, and resources and thus find solutions to help master the difficult and unfamiliar in other environments (Hattie, Marsh, Neill, & Richards, 1997). While some people can learn by sitting and listening, most learn best when all five of their senses are engaged. When the emphasis is on "doing," the lessons tend to be more memorable, the messages more enduring (Smolowe, Butler, Murray, 1999). While adventure activities are often outfitted with playful, memorable props, the real business of these activities revolves around eliciting authentic behaviors that serve to provide a rich exploration of human nature. Through the constant probing, dissecting and debriefing that accompanies each activity, a learning community begins to emerge that then builds on itself, paving the way for ever-deeper exploration (Smolowe, Butler, Murray, 1999).

In summary, experiential therapies have been around for centuries but have not been termed as such. More recently, **experiential therapy** is defined as viewing any hands-on activity as experiential and therapeutic because one is "experiencing" the event or situation and learning from the experience. In the past, the most familiar experiential therapies were wilderness therapy and ropes courses. More recently, Equine-Assisted Psychotherapy (EAP) has been added to that list of therapies incorporating experiential methodology.

Various Methods to Experiential Learning

In an authentic adventure environment, activities serve as a springboard to lead from engagement to exploration to enlightenment. Whether the challenge is improving relationships (either internally or externally), reinforcing values, examining leadership and/or personality styles, identifying norms or building more effective teams, adventure is a potent tool for exploring, learning, discussing, sharing and all of these are important precursors to sustainable change (Smolowe, Butler, Murray, 1999).

Outdoor-adventure therapy benefits include an improvement in interpersonal and cognitive problem-solving skills (Walton, 1985), a reduction in problem behaviors (Pommier, 1994), and an increase in self-efficacy and self-esteem (Hughes, 1993). Used effectively, adventure becomes a key for unlocking closed minds, stimulating fresh thinking, encouraging meaningful dialogue, and triggering learning that is transferable to life. Removed from familiar surroundings and presented with challenges where participants know neither what to expect nor what is expected of them, they are free simply to participate. According to Smolowe, Butler, & Murray (1999), an experiential activity then "holds up a mirror to reflect back information about personal styles, modes of interaction, options, choices and potential. Of the many paths that lead to knowledge, doing is the route that leaves the most vivid and enduring impression." As a result, experiential activities help people to respond proactively rather than reactively to therapy (Smolowe, et. al, 1999).

Wilderness Therapy

Experiential approaches, such as wilderness therapy as depicted in Figure 1.1, are conducive to the physical and emotional growth of each person involved. For instance, living in the outdoors for an extended period of time provides opportunities for all to play and work together, with just enough rules to ensure safety. Being involved in organizing, planning, and supervising activities related to their own welfare, participants come to recognize the values of cooperative, collective effort. Not only do they develop a sense of responsibility for their own actions, but they come to recognize that their decisions often affect the health and welfare of the rest of the group (Ledlie, 1951). Inevitably, surviving in the wilderness creates minor stresses and strains, which give participants the opportunity to problem-solve and achieve success. By succeeding in handling small crises, participants feel more confident and competent when larger crises arise in their lives (Ledlie, 1951).

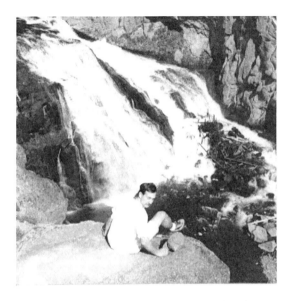

**Figure 1.1
Wilderness Therapy**

Task given is to climb down from the cliff's edge to the bottom of the waterfall.

Consequently, the therapeutic changes occur because wilderness evokes coping behaviors rather than defensive behaviors. It is a difficult, natural, or healthful environment experience and the opportunity to interact with and/or observe animals and plants, which in itself has been found to be therapeutic (Levitt, 1994). Through wilderness therapy, these experiences are used as opportunities for facilitating significant growth (Cole, Erdman, & Rothblum, 1994).

The primitive nature of a wilderness experience seems to help strip life down to its very essentials. In the wilderness, circumstances can be demanding, consequences are immediate, and facades are often quickly discarded. This experience provides the counselor with an unparalleled vantage point for assessment, instruction, intervention, and application around therapeutic concerns (Kehler, 1998). Wilderness therapy deliberately makes use of the healing effect of natural, wilderness setting (Davis-Berman & Berman, 1994). In this setting, although rock climbing or river rafting might be presented, the main intention is to provide clients with opportunities to make contact with the meanings and consequences derived from engaging in this experience over an extended amount of time. During this time, they confront natural challenges presented by weather, fatigue or physical objects such as rivers and mountains. Clients see clearly the ways in which nature and life parallel. The fact that nature can be unforgiving and punishing, as well as inspiring and rewarding, provides profound teaching without judgment or interpretation (Peel & Richards, 2005).

Ropes Course

A **ropes course,** as depicted in Figure 1.2, is a series of low and high element challenges created with obstacles and ropes designed to create an environment that stretches people physically, intellectually, emotionally, and spiritually. A ropes course experience, like wilderness therapy, presents opportunities for participants to explore their fears, build trust in themselves and others, and try out their leadership skills within a safe and supportive environment (Stopha, 1994). Human (2006) quotes Greyling Viljoen who states:

> *The goal of using ropes courses is to take people out of their comfort zone and place them into their stretch zone, but not into their panic zone. People experience discomfort and vulnerability in their stretch zone and it is here where the potential for personal growth lies.*

Ropes courses help clients become more aware of their own anxieties. A ropes course creates an opportunity for their anxiety to come into awareness— identifying triggers as well as strategies used to deal with anxiety. This process of awareness aids in personal growth (Human, 2006). Most of the exercises involve a combination of mental problem solving and physical challenge. The emphasis is on both personal growth and team collaboration (Kehler, 1998).

Discussions can cover topics of leadership, following, styles of communication, how the group handles suggestions from others, feelings about the end result, as well as topics specific to the concerns of the participants. Reflection on the implications of the activity to "real life" is also an important part of the debriefing process (Stopha, 1994). Clearly, the personal, social, emotional, and cognitive benefits of ropes courses include enhancing self-concept, confidence, and self-esteem; improving social, school/work, and attitudes and behavior; decreasing pathological symptoms; enhancing relations; and improving quality and quantity of interactions (Levitt, 1994).

Figure 1.2 High Ropes Course

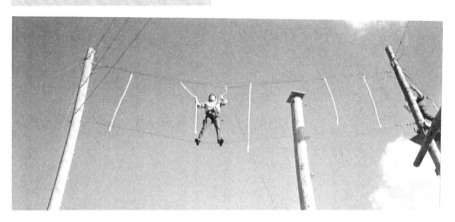

Equine-Assisted Psychotherapy

Equine-Assisted Psychotherapy (EAP) incorporates horses experientially for emotional growth and learning. EAP encompasses many of the same components and benefits as the previously mentioned experiential approaches with the added dimension of dealing with large, live animals. This unique component adds another relational dimension to this formula increasing the therapeutic benefit. According to Equine-Assisted Growth and Learning Association (EAGALA, 2006, 2012), it is a collaborative effort between a licensed therapist and a horse professional working with the clients and horses to address treatment goals. In EAP, clients learn about themselves and others by participating in activities with the horses, and then discussing thoughts, beliefs, behaviors, and patterns. EAP is a powerfully effective tool in assisting participants who are fearful, anxious, depressed, angry, dissociative, or who have a variety of other emotional challenges. Introducing therapeutic work with the horse to a person who is accustomed to conventional "office therapy" is, in itself, a change. Introducing horses into the session breaks through the participant's defensive barriers and requires him/her to develop fresh insights and new perspectives from old relationships and behavior patterns (Tyler, 1994).

An initial positive experience with a horse may be utilized as a springboard toward other experiences, which foster feelings of self-confidence and an improved ability to relate and to communicate with others (Tyler, 1994). The lulling rhythm of the horse's movement combined with the sights, scents, and sounds of natural surroundings within the arena elevates the spirit, alleviates tension, and may be used as an adjunct or an introduction to more conversational forms of therapy and visual imagery in the office (Tyler, 1994).

EAP also evolves naturally and very easily for the therapist using horses as "co-facilitators." Elements of teamwork, cooperation, communication, successful challenge, healthy competition and improved socialization are all easily introduced and coordinated, using the horse as a medium (Tyler, 1994). Each activity is designed with a specific objective and underlying theme. The dynamics brought out by the activity are discussed in the debriefing. As summarized by Ham, Lawrence, and Tucker (1998), EAP offers many unique advantages: (1) the opportunity to work with a live animal adds a valuable dynamic to relationship interaction, (2) participants build confidence and self-esteem and learn responsibility while caring for an animal, and (3) participants learn to develop an awareness of equine body-language that relates to human body language and communication.

The horse is the key to separating EAP from other forms of experiential therapies. According to EAGALA (2006), if an activity is conducted that could be equally effective without the horse, it isn't truly EAP. EAP is about the horses doing the work of effecting change in people's lives, and it is about the interactions between the client and the horse that are significant (EAGALA, 2006). Just as in other experiential therapies, the facilitators are there to provide the opportunities and bring awareness to the lessons being learned.

Horses are honest teachers with personalities as varied as those of humans, and therefore they react differently to each person and each action. How the animal responds to the participant's behavior offers immediate feedback. This response helps to develop and promote many qualities such as empathy, assertiveness, leadership, open-mindedness, thought, endurance, and patience (Ham et al., 1998). The relaxed yet supportive setting also promotes accountability, a sense of belonging, as well as the importance of group effort and accomplishment (Ham et al., 1998).The issues raised and the techniques used to manage the horse's behavior will help teach the participant skills needed for his/her own practical life application. This translates to other areas of therapy, enabling the participant to relate more openly (Ham et al., 1998).

Equine-Assisted Psychotherapy includes a sequence of interactive horse activities/experiences for the purpose of goal setting, awareness, trust, group problem-solving, individual problem-solving, and processing/transfer. Through the use of these experiences, EAP counselors seek to assist participants in the development of insight and skills that transfer to their lives after they have completed the activities. Without such positive transfer, therapy can have limited long-term value (Luckner & Nadler, 1995).

With experiential therapies such as EAP, the process—how they handle the experience—is more valuable than the content. Witman (1993) suggested that "the integration of interpersonal and human relations skills such as the understanding of group dynamics, building a climate of trust within a group, knowing how to stimulate motivation, and interpreting nonverbal expressions" (p. 48) are essential skills experiential therapists must incorporate for the participants to gain long-term benefits. The mission of experiential therapy as used in EAP is to use horses, activity, and recreation to help people deal with problems that serve as barriers and to assist them in growing toward their highest level of health and wellness.

Equine-Assisted Psychotherapy focuses on the nature of the animals which helps remove the intensity of a participants' anxieties and allows them to relax into the present. Often, opening up to nature allows the shift in focus necessary for the subconscious mind to take over and solve the problems that loom so powerfully over them and through which logic has not shown them a clear way. Nature may lead them to the answers that they had within them all along. Being in and with nature, particularly horses, helps attune the participants to the fact that they are not separate beings, but are related to and influenced by their surroundings. This experience can reduce feelings of alienation and unacceptability and bring them back to feeling more connected with others and even more relieved, loved, and accepted as demonstrated in Figure 1.3 (Angell, 1994).

Figure 1.3 -- EAP activity brings people together increasing sense of belonging and significance in relationships.

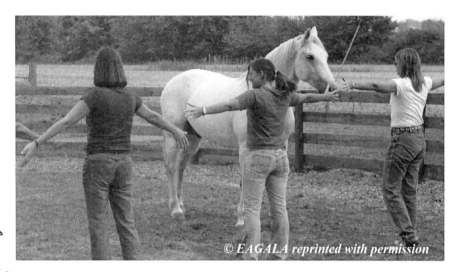

© EAGALA reprinted with permission

Rhoades (1972) argued that the most compelling reason for using horses in their natural environment is that it requires certain responses which are of value: "cooperation, clear thinking and planning, careful observation, resourcefulness, persistence and adaptability....These responses are not demanded by the environment, but rather the manner in which the program forces students to interact with the environment" (p. 26).

Another reason for the use of horses as a therapeutic intervention is the value of using adventure activities with a horse to increase participants' self esteem, alter their locus of control, reduce antisocial behavior, and improve problem solving abilities (Luckner & Nadler, 1995).

Through Equine-Assisted Psychotherapy, participants will begin to regain their equilibrium disrupted by stressors so that they may once again resume their quest for actualization within this supportive and non-threatening atmosphere. Oftentimes, participants have fun as they learn new skills, new behaviors, new ways to interact with each other, new philosophies and values, and new cognition about themselves. In short, they learn that they can be successful in their interactions with each other (Austin, 1998). EAP provides a context in which they can learn, interact, express individualism, and self-actualize, while deepening existing relationships (Stumbo & Peterson, 1998).

Equine-Assisted Psychotherapy can be free from constraint. EAP involves intrinsic motivation and provides an opportunity for participants to experience a tremendous amount of control in their lives. EAP permits them to suspend everyday rules and conventions in order to "be themselves" and "let their hair down" (Austin, 1998). The establishment and fulfillment of personal and group goals in outdoor physical activities, the group experience, and the opportunity to experience and master stressful situations as a group are all important components of EAP (Hattie et al., 1997).

Benefits of Processing

The long-term benefits to EAP and other experiential approaches depend highly on the **processing** -- talking about what is going on. Experiential therapies such as EAP can serve as a metaphor for the life of the participants as the session's experiences can clarify real-life situations and thereby help the participants contend with them (Miles, 1993). Processing can occur prior to, during, or after the adventure experience. In EAP, processing activities are used to: (a) help participants focus or increase their awareness of issues prior to an event or the entire experience; (b) facilitate awareness or promote change while an experience is occurring; (c) reflect, analyze, describe, or discuss an experience after it is completed; and/or (d) reinforce perceptions of change and promote integration in their lives after the experience is completed (Gass, 1993a). Clearly, experience and research alike indicate that therapeutic recreation with process included, as conducted in EAP, has particularly strong, lasting effects (Hattie et al., 1997).

In Equine-Assisted Psychotherapy, participants are encouraged to reflect and express the thoughts and feelings that they are experiencing. Awareness of what they specifically did thought, and felt prior to a breakthrough or retreat should be emphasized. Processing is essential if there is going to be generalization and transfer (Nadler, 1993). A goal of EAP is to assist participants in forming their own linkages to what they are learning. This allows participants to integrate their new knowledge and desired behavior with their lifestyle during the remainder of their time and continue with these changes when they get back home (Nadler, 1993). An underlying assumption of this philosophy is that insight and awareness into the nature of problems does not produce positive change by itself. Change can best occur from process of translating insight into action through the active experiencing of new situations as EAP demonstrates (Clapp & Rudolph, 1993).

One of the primary purposes of experiential therapy, specifically equine-assisted activities, is to assist people in developing insight and skills that transfer to their lives. Without such positive transfer, activities such as EAP have limited long-term value. The role of the counseling team in facilitating meaningful exchanges of insights, thoughts, feelings, reactions, and the co-constructing of new stories is a delicate and complex one (Luckner & Nadler, 1995).

By allowing the treatment team to actually observe their clients attempting to solve problems, experiential therapy can help everyone involved better understand and recognize their patterns of relating. Experiential therapies, such as EAP, offer more than the opportunity for assessment; they offer life-changing experiences as well (Kehler, 1998). White (1992) summarizes EAP's contributions by saying, "The stories that we enter into with our experience have real effects on our lives. The expression of our experience through these stories shapes or makes-up our lives and our relationships (p. 81). It is these metaphorical stories that are so vital to the lasting impact of the EAP experience. In some ways, metaphors are the most important protectors of people. When all else fails, there are always memories and stories. They can transcend time and distance, poverty and ill health. These metaphors of food, places, animals, trips, beloved objects and beloved people become the connecting tissue of people. They give people's lives a context and meaning, a history and philosophy (White, 1992).

Topics for Discussion:

1. *What is experiential therapy and identify various forms of experiential methods? Discuss.*

2. *Discuss the advantages and disadvantages to experiential therapy over traditional therapy.*

3. *Discuss scenarios or situations when experiential therapy might not be an appropriate fit for the client. Give examples.*

4. *What makes experiential learning so effective?*

5. *Share a personal experiential activity or experience and why it was so meaningful to you.*

6. *Define and discuss the difference between content and process in relation to a counseling session.*

Chapter Notes

CHAPTER 1

Chapter Notes

2 KEY THEORETICAL ORIENTATIONS

Objectives:

- **Describe five primary theories behind the Equine-Assisted Psychotherapy approach**
- **Discuss the therapist's role in each approach**
- **Explore the benefits each theory contributes to Equine-Assisted Psychotherapy**

In this chapter, you will examine the five main theories behind the methodology of Equine-Assisted Psychotherapy (EAP). Each of the various theories has unique and significant contributions to the effectiveness of EAP. As you read through the five primary theories, keep in mind that other theories can be incorporated depending on the therapist's orientation and/or the client's needs. Nevertheless, the five theories discussed in this chapter are the most widely used and fundamental within the therapeutic paradigm of Equine-Assisted Psychotherapy.

Cognitive-Behavioral Theory

View of Human Nature

Cognitive-Behavior Theory, also known as rational-emotive behavior therapy (REBT), is based on the assumption that human beings are born with a potential for both rational, or straight, thinking and irrational, or crooked, thinking. People have predispositions to self-preservation, happiness, thinking and verbalizing, loving, communion with others, and growth and self-actualization. They also have propensities for self-destruction, avoidance of thought, procrastination, endless repetition of mistakes, superstition, intolerance, perfectionism and self-blame, and avoidance of actualizing growth potentials. Taking for granted that humans are fallible, REBT attempts to help them accept themselves as creatures who will continue to make mistakes yet at the same time learn to live more at peace with themselves (Ellis & Dryden, 1987; Corey, 2009). Ellis has concluded that humans are self-talking, self-evaluating, and self-sustaining. They develop emotional and behavioral difficulties when they take simple preferences (desires for love, approval, success) and make the mistake of thinking of them as dire needs. Ellis also affirms that humans have inborn tendencies toward growth and actualization, yet they often sabotage their movement toward growth as a result of their inborn tendency toward crooked thinking and also the self-defeating patterns they have learned (Ellis & Dryden, 1987).

A-B-C- Theory of Personality

As REBT contests, emotional disturbances are largely the product of irrational, self-defeating thinking. So, in REBT, the client and the therapist work together to dispute the irrational beliefs that are causing disturbed emotional consequences. They work toward transforming an unrealistic, immature, demanding, and absolutist style of thinking into a realistic, mature, logical, and empirical approach to thinking and behaving. This transformation results in more appropriate feeling and reactions to life's situations (Kottler & Shepard, 2011). The following diagram will clarify the interaction of the various components being discussed (Corey, 1996, 2009):

A (activating event) ← B (belief) → C (emotional and behavioral consequence)
↑
D (disputing intervention) → E (effect) → F (new feeling)

In sum, philosophical restructuring to change our dysfunctional personality involves the following steps: (1) fully acknowledging that we are largely responsible for creating our own emotional problems, (2) accepting the notion that we have the ability to change these disturbances significantly, (3) recognizing that our emotional problems largely stem from irrational beliefs, and (4) clearly perceiving these beliefs, (5) seeing the value of disputing such foolish beliefs, using rigorous methods, (6) accepting the fact that if we expect to change, we had better work hard in emotive and behavioral ways to counteract our beliefs and the dysfunctional feelings and actions that follow, and (7) practicing REBT methods of uprooting or changing disturbed consequences for the rest of our life (Ellis, 1988, 2001, 2002; Corey, 2009).

Therapist's Function and Role

A therapist who works within this framework functions differently from most other practitioners. Because REBT is essentially a cognitive and directive behavioral process, it often minimizes the intense relationship between the therapist and the client. The therapist mainly employs a persuasive methodology that emphasizes education. Ellis (1992) outlines what the REBT practitioner does:

- encourages clients to discover a few basic irrational ideas that motivate much disturbed behavior
- challenges clients to validate their ideas
- demonstrates to clients the illogical nature of their thinking
- uses a logical analysis to minimize these irrational beliefs
- shows how these beliefs are inoperative and how they will lead to future emotional and behavioral disturbances
- explains how these ideas can be replaced with more rational ideas that are empirically grounded
- teaches clients how to apply the scientific approach to thinking so that they can observe and minimize present or future irrational ideas and illogical deductions that foster self-destructive ways of feeling and behaving
- uses several cognitive, emotive, and behavioral methods to help clients work directly on their feelings and to act against their disturbances

Reality Therapy

View of Human Nature

Reality Therapy, also known as Control Theory and/or Choice Theory, rests on the notion that human behavior is purposeful and originates completely from within the individual rather than from external forces. Although environmental factors have an influence on our decisions, our behavior is not caused by them. All of our internally motivated behavior is geared toward getting things we want that satisfy one or more of our basic human needs. Glasser (1985, 1989) identifies these as the four psychological needs for belonging, power, freedom, and fun and the one physiological need for survival (Corey, 2009). Control theory explains that our brain functions as a control system to get us what we want to satisfy these needs. Although we all possess the same five needs, each of us fulfills them in unique ways. We develop an inner "picture album" of specific wants, also called a "quality world," which contains precise images of how we would best like to fulfill our needs (Corey, 2009). A major goal of reality therapy is to teach people better and more effective ways of attaining what they want in life.

Explanation of Behavior

Glasser (1989) explains the concept of total behavior by comparing how we function to how a car functions (Corey, 2009; Wubbolding, 2011). Just as the four wheels guide a car, so do the four components of our total behavior influence our direction in life. Wubbolding (2011) describes these components of total behavior as:

- **Doing** meaning actions or active behaviors such as getting up and going to work
- **Thinking** which is generating thoughts and self-statements
- **Feelings** such as anger, joy, pain, depression, and anxiety
- **Physiology** which is how the body responds, such as sweating or developing psychosomatic symptoms

Although these behavioral components always blend to make a whole or total behavior, they can be distinguished from one another, and one of them is usually more prominent than the others (Glasser, 1989).

When explaining the concept of total behavior as portrayed in Figure 2.1, Glasser (1992) gives emphasis to the "two front wheels" (doing and thinking), which steer us, just as the front wheels steer the direction of a car. It is difficult to directly change how we are feeling, separately from what we are doing or thinking. However, we have an almost complete ability to change what we are doing and thinking, in spite of how we might be feeling:

> *In reality therapy, we focus on helping other people to choose or change the only parts they can change, which are their actions and thoughts. It is not that we ignore or deny feelings and/or physiology; it is that we do not dwell upon what no one can change directly (p. 7).*

To summarize, reality theory asserts that all we ever do from birth to death is behave, and every total behavior is always our best attempt to get what we want to satisfy our needs. In this context, behavior is purposeful because it is designed to close the gap between what we want and what we perceive that we are getting.

Figure 2.1. Reality Theory Total Behavior Car

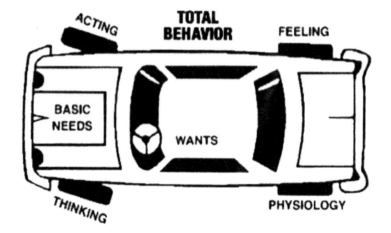

Characteristics of Reality Therapy

Reality Therapy has consistently emphasized **responsibility**, which Glasser (1992) defines as behavior that satisfies one's needs in ways that do not interfere with others fulfilling their needs. Responsible people are autonomous in the sense that they know what they want from life and make plans for meeting their needs and goals. In short, responsibility means that people have learned to take effective control of their lives.

Reality therapists believe that the client is responsible for the choices they make. This theory changes the focus of responsibility to choice and choosing to the client. Reality therapists deal with people "as if" they have choices. Therapists focus on those areas where clients have choice, for doing so gets them closer to the people they need (Corey, 2009).

Reality therapy sees transference as a way for the therapist to remain hidden as a person. Transference is defined and discussed further in Chapters 14 and 17. Glasser calls for therapists to be themselves and not to think or teach that they are playing the role of the client's mother or father. The reality therapist deals with whatever perceptions clients have, and there is no attempt to teach clients that their reactions and views are other than what they state. Instead of dwelling on a client's past failures, reality therapists look to the past for evidences of the client's ability to successfully control the world, and they help clients deal with situations that are directly related to their present lives (Glasser, 1992; Corey, 2009).

Reality therapists consistently attempt to focus clients on what they are doing now. They also avoid discussing clients' feeling or physiology as though these were separate from their total behavior (Corey, 2009). Counselors help their clients see connections between what they are feeling and their concurrent actions and thoughts. Although reality therapists focus on the actions and thoughts of clients (the front wheels that drive the car), they consider it quite legitimate to talk about feelings and physiology. When people begin to act differently, they will also begin to feel differently.

Reality therapy holds that punishment is not a useful means of changing behavior. Instead of being punished, individuals can learn to accept the reasonable consequences that flow from their actions. By not making critical comments, by refusing to accept excuses, and by remaining nonjudgmental, counselors are in a position to ask clients if they are really interested in changing (Glasser, 1992).

Therapist's Function in Therapy

Reality therapists challenge clients with the basic question of reality therapy, "Is what you are choosing to do getting you what you want?" If clients make the judgment that what they are doing is not working, therapists may suggest an alternative course of action (Glasser, 1989; Kottler & Shepard, 2011). The counselor also teaches clients how they can create a "success identity" by accepting accountability for their own chosen behaviors (Glasser, 1986). This role requires counselors to perform several functions:

- ➢ establishing a structure and limits for the sessions

- establishing rapport based on care and respect
- focusing on the individual's strengths and potentials that can lead to success
- actively promoting discussion of the client's current behavior and actively discouraging excuses for irresponsible or ineffective behavior
- introducing and fostering the process of evaluating realistically attainable wants
- teaching clients to formulate and carry out plans to change their behaviors
- helping clients find ways to meet their needs and encouraging them not to give up easily, even if they become discouraged

Gestalt Therapy

Gestalt counseling is an experiential therapy stressing here-and-now awareness. According to Kottler & Shepard (2011), the major focus of gestalt therapy is on the "what" and "how" of behavior and the role of unfinished business from the past that prevents effective functioning in the present. A central therapeutic aim is to challenge the client to move more fully into self-support. In this approach, the therapist assists clients to experience all feelings more fully, and this enables them to make their own interpretations. The therapist avoids making interpretations and instead focuses on how clients are behaving. Clients identify their own unfinished business, and they work through the blockages impeding their growth. They do this largely by re-experiencing past situations as though they were happening in the present. Therapists have many techniques at their disposal, all of which have two things in common: they are designed to intensify direct experiencing and to integrate conflicting feelings (Corey, 1996).

View of Human Nature

The Gestalt view of human nature is rooted in existential philosophy. Genuine knowledge is the product of what is immediately evident in the experience of the perceiver. Therapy aims not at analysis but at integration of sometimes conflicting dimensions within the person. The process of "re-owning" parts of oneself that have been disowned and the unification process proceed step by step until clients become strong enough to carry on with their own personal growth. By becoming aware, they become able to make informed choices and thus to live a meaningful existence. A basic assumption of Gestalt therapy is that individuals can deal with their life problems themselves, especially if they are fully aware of what is happening in and around them. Because of certain problems in development, people find various ways to avoid problems and, therefore, reach impasses in their personal growth. The Gestalt theory of change posits that the more we attempt to be whom or what we are not, the more we remain the same (Corey, 1996, 2009). According to Beisser's (1970) paradoxical theory of change, we change when we become aware of what we are, as opposed to trying to become what we are not. What is important is for clients to be as fully as possible in their current position, rather than striving to become what they "should be" (Corey, 2009).

A concept related to unfinished business is avoidance, which refers to the means people use to keep themselves from facing unfinished business and from experiencing the uncomfortable emotions associated with unfinished situations. Because we have a tendency to avoid confronting and fully experiencing our anxiety, grief, guilt, and other uncomfortable emotions, the emotions become a nagging undercurrent that prevents us from being fully alive (Kottler & Shepard, 2011). Thus, the Gestalt therapist encourages expressing in the now of the therapeutic session intense feelings never directly expressed before. By going beyond our avoidances, we make it possible to dispose of unfinished business that interferes with our present life, and we move toward health and integration (Corey, 1996).

Therapeutic Goals

The basic goal of Gestalt therapy is attaining awareness and, with it, greater choice and responsibility. Awareness includes knowing the environment, knowing oneself, accepting oneself, and being able to make contact with others (Corey, 1996, 2009).

Through a creative involvement in Gestalt process, clients will:

- move toward increased awareness of themselves
- gradually assume ownership of their experience (as opposed to making others responsible for what they are thinking, feeling, and doing)

- ➤ develop skills and acquire values that will allow them to satisfy their needs without violating the rights of others
- ➤ become more aware of all of their senses
- ➤ learn to accept responsibility for what they do, including accepting the consequences of their actions
- ➤ move from outside support toward increasing internal support
- ➤ be able to ask for and get help from others and give to others (Zinker, 1978).

Gestalt therapists notice what is in both the foreground and the background. They focus on the client's feelings, awareness at the moment, body messages, energy, avoidance, and blocks to awareness. An important function of the Gestalt therapist is paying attention to the client's body language. These nonverbal cues provide rich information, because they often betray feelings of which the client is unaware (Corey, 1996, 2009). Perls (1969) writes that a client's posture, movements, gestures, voice, hesitations, and other cues tell the real story. He warns that verbal communication is usually a lie and that if therapists are content-oriented, they miss the essence of the person. Real communication is beyond words.

Gestalt therapy uses confrontation therapeutically. **Confrontation** can be done in such a way that clients cooperate, especially when they are invited to examine their behaviors, attitudes, and thoughts. Gestalt therapists encourage clients to look at certain incongruities, especially gaps between verbal and nonverbal communication (Corey, 2009).

Gestalt therapy emphasizes the importance of a therapist learning how to listen to the metaphors of clients. By paying attention to metaphors, the therapist gets rich clues to a client's internal struggles.

Brief Therapy

You can call it focused, short-term, strategic, solution-oriented, cost-effective, time-effective, time-limited, time-sensitive, or just plain old brief therapy (Oliver, Hasz, Richburg, 1997). A simple definition isn't as easy as you might think. It can't be defined merely in terms of number of sessions, length of sessions, or total time elapsed between the first and the last sessions. At its core, brief therapy is a way of thinking about change as much as a way of helping people change. The bottom-

CHAPTER 2

line goals are helping clients overcome the difficulties that are keeping them from functioning in healthy ways and, in the process, giving them new ways to handle future problems in a more effective manner (Oliver, Hasz, Richburg, 1997; Corey, 2009; Kottler & Shepard, 2011).

According to researchers Koss and Butcher (1986), most brief therapists strive to accomplish one or more of the following goals: removal or improvement of the patient's most disabling symptoms as rapidly as possible, prompt reestablishment of the patient's previous emotional equilibrium, and development of the patient's understanding of the current disturbance and increased coping ability in the future.

Ideally, therapy is brief and intermittent throughout the life cycle and is needed at times when old defenses no longer suffice, and the client is most receptive to change. Brief therapy is more than just a set of clever techniques or compacted long-term therapy. One of the most effective ways to differentiate brief therapies from long-term therapies is to examine the underlying assumptions of each approach (Oliver, Hasz, Richburg, 1997).

Table 2.1 is a modified and edited version of Budman and Gurman's (1983) original sixteen core assumptions of brief versus long-term therapy. Read through the following list of fourteen assumptions and put a check by the statements that most reflect your practice and make you the most comfortable.

If the majority of your checks were next to the odd-numbered statements, you are probably most comfortable with long-term therapy. If more of your checks are next to the even-numbered statements, you are more comfortable with brief therapy (Oliver, Hasz, Richburg, 1997).

After a thorough review of a wide range of the brief-therapy literature, Oliver, Hasz, and Richburg (1997) have identified seven key assumptions that distinguish most brief therapies.

Table 2.1 Principles of Brief versus Long-term Therapy

- 1. Seeks change in basic character.
- 2. Prefers practical, most concise, and least radical intervention and does not believe in notion of "cure."
- 3. Believes that significant psychological change is unlikely in everyday life.
- 4. Maintains an adult development perspective from which significant psychological change is viewed as inevitable.
- 5. Sees presenting problem as reflecting a more pervasive underlying pathology.
- 6. Emphasizes patient's strengths and resources; presenting problems are taken seriously, although not necessarily at face value.
- 7. Believes the therapist needs to be there as patient makes significant changes.
- 8. Accepts that many changes will occur after therapy and will not be observable to the therapist.
- 9. Sees therapy as having a timeless quality and is patient and willing to wait for change.
- 10. Does not accept the timelessness of some models of therapy.
- 11. Views psychotherapy as almost always benign and useful.
- 12. Views psychotherapy as sometimes useful and sometimes harmful.
- 13. Sees the patient's being in therapy as one of the most important parts of patient's life.
- 14. Sees the patient's being in the world as more important than being in therapy.

Specific Treatment Goals

Brief therapists believe that the focus needs to be clarified from the very beginning. Our job as a brief therapist is to negotiate solvable problems and realistic treatment goals.

Along this line, Mann and Goldman (1973) write:

> *It is long been my conviction that long-term psychotherapy with insufficiently or inaccurately defined treatment goals leads to a steady widening of and diffusion of content. This creates a growing sense of ambiguity in the mind of the therapist as to what he is about, and, while it may affect the patient similarly, it surely increases the patient's dependence on the therapist. The result is that patient and therapist*

come to need each other, so that bringing the case to a conclusion seems impossible. Since treatment is the responsibility of the therapist, the problem of excessively long treatment lies in the domain of the therapist and not the patient. Further, it has been some brief therapists' position that the constant exposure to large doses of severe psychopathology that is a rather natural consequence of training programs in psychiatry tends to diminish the young therapist's peripheral vision, so to speak, so that he is unable to appreciate the assets of the patient before him. He tends to develop very little confidence in his patient's ability, capacity, and motivation to help himself. It is a short step then to being convinced that no patient can long survive without his close and indefinitely prolonged attention.

Brief therapy is focused. The challenge isn't how brief we can make it. The challenge is to identify the need and then clarify what can and can't be accomplished in this episode of treatment with the resources that are available. At a later time, you can move on to another focus (Oliver, Hasz, Richburg, 1997).

Focused Use of Time

Traditional approaches to psychotherapy are based on the assumption that the presenting problem is not the real problem but merely a symptom of a much deeper psychological or interpersonal problem that must be uncovered, interpreted, and worked through. These approaches assume that real change takes place through an understanding of the problem and a focus on it. In order to be effective, therapy must be intensive, reconstructive, and time-consuming (Oliver, Hasz, Richburg, 1997).

Effective brief therapy involves a rapid assessment and integration of assessment within treatment. The past can be acknowledged in the context of moving on in the present, but the emphasis is on intervening in the present. We want clients to take away from the session something that is useful, helpful, and beneficial to them. This involves frequently reviewing progress and discarding ineffective interventions (Oliver, Hasz, Richburg, 1997).

According to de Shazer (1991), brief therapy simply means therapy that takes as few sessions as possible for you to develop a satisfactory solution. At any given time any client has a variety of concerns and problems that might be helpful to discuss in a counseling context. However, the focus of brief therapy is the problem or issue that is keeping the person stuck and hindering him or her from functioning in healthy ways.

Brief therapists find it helpful to emphasize the direction of change rather than the magnitude of change. More is not necessarily better. We ask clients what, where, and how, rather than how much (Oliver, Hasz, Richburg, 1997).

Use of Techniques

Some therapists assume that whatever the clients' needs are, they will fit into one correct theoretical mold. The best therapy listens to the needs of the clients and shapes the therapy to meet those needs. While the goal of change for two people may be similar, the pathways to that goal may be significantly different. An intervention that is effective for one client may be absolutely useless for another. The best brief therapists have a variety of tools in their therapeutic toolbox (Oliver, Hasz, Richburg, 1997).

A State of Mind

Brief therapy is rarely officially terminated. Rather it is interrupted, and the client is encouraged to return if, in future life stages or traumas, another episode of therapy would be helpful. While dealing with the presenting problem, there is an opportunity to address subsequent problems. However, there is no belief that the course of this person's life will not lead to a future problem that could benefit from treatment (Oliver, Hasz, Richburg, 1997).

Another, and we believe a much more realistic model, is to look to the doctor-patient relationship in medicine. If you go to see your family practice physician and receive successful treatment for a particular virus, it doesn't mean that you will never have to deal with that virus again for the rest of your life. It does mean that when you return for another visit, both you and the doctor will remember the symptoms and be able to much more quickly identify the treatment that worked (Oliver, Hasz, Richburg, 1997).

Emphasis on Strengths and Resources

Some therapists have a tendency to look for and focus on shortcomings, symptoms, defense mechanisms, syndromes, and dynamics. When looking through these lenses, counselors could rate a successfully functioning person as "sick." However, the brief therapist has an orientation to health or strength rather than to sickness or weakness.
To summarize this perspective, Saleeby (1992) wrote:

> *At the very least, the strengths perspective obligates workers to understand that, however downtrodden or sick, individuals have survived (and in some cases even thrived). They have taken steps, summoned up resources, and coped. We need to know what they have done, how they have done it, what they have learned from doing it, and what resources (inner and outer) were available in their struggle to surmount their troubles. People are always working on their situations, even if just deciding to be resigned to them; as helpers we must tap into that work, elucidate it, find and build on its possibilities (p. 171).*

Small Changes are Significant

One key assumption of brief therapy is that small changes can be, and often are, significant. In Fisch, Weakland, & Segal's foreword to *The Tactics of Change (1982),* Milton Erickson is quoted saying,

> *Psychotherapy is sought not primarily for enlightenment about the unchangeable past but because of the dissatisfaction with the present and a desire to better the future. In what direction and how much change is needed neither the patient nor the therapist can know. But a change in the current situation is required, and once established, however small, necessitates other minor changes, and a snowballing effect of these minor changes leads to other more significant changes in accord with the patient's potentials.*

Systems Theory

The systems perspective holds particular importance for the social institution of the family. As a systems theorist, the therapist recognizes that an individual's actions cannot be understood separately from his/her interactions with other members of the family. This theory holds true for any group structure. Family therapists recognize that the context of social interactions between members plays a major role in determining each individual's behavior. They also recognize that if change occurs in one person, it will affect every other family member (Gass, 1993b; Corey, 2009; Kottler & Shepard, 2011).

Therapeutic Process of Change

It often happens that when people struggle in their attempts to produce desired changes to problems, they find that their solutions maintain, reinforce, or even exacerbate the issues. This is especially true when problems are difficult or maintained by a destructive pattern or cycle (Nadler, 1993). In attempting to find answers to this troublesome phenomenon, Watzlawick, Weakland, and Fisch (1974) have stated that random events, followed by their unexpected, unusual, repetitious "more of the same" efforts have failed.

Table 2.2 Principles of Therapy in Systems Theory

> People consist of individual learners, always actively searching for and constructing new meanings, always learning.
> The process of learning is self-regulating and self-preserving.
> Knowledge consists of past constructions.
> The best predictor of what and how a family will learn is what they already know.
> Learning often proceeds from whole to part of whole.
> Errors are critical to learning.
> Meaningful learning occurs through reflection and resolution of cognitive conflict and thus serves to negate earlier, incomplete levels of understanding.
> People learn best from experiences which they are passionately interested and involved in.
> People learn best from people they trust.

One of the cornerstones of systems theory is the encouragement of groups to do things they might not ordinarily do; to leave their safe, familiar, comfortable, and predictable world and enter into uncomfortable new territory. In doing so, unique answers or outcomes may emerge (White & Epston, 1990). Not only is this style of therapy new for most people, but so are the emotions, thoughts, and interactions that accompany these experiences. Members may feel awkward, unfamiliar, and at risk as they move into areas that are unknown to them. The task of the counseling team is to help people enter into these areas so that positive change and resulting growth can occur (Nadler, 1993).

Personal Choice and Responsibility

Systems theory embraces the notion that each person has the responsibility for his/her own actions and the capacity for making self-directed and wise choices regarding their behavior (Austin, 1998). Systems theory recognizes that people have the capacity for self-development throughout their lives. A key assumption is that each of them has a need to grow and to realize their full potential (Austin, 1998). Murphy (1975) believes that systems therapists must seek "to promote the capacity and ability of groups and individuals to make self-determined and responsible choices – in light of their needs to grow, to explore new possibilities, and to realize their full potentials" (p. 2).

Constructing New Meaning

Fundamental to the systems theory perspective is the tenet that people learn by making sense of what is experienced. According to the system theory approach to therapy, there is the "search for the exception," when the problem does not exist, (de Shazer, 1988) or the "unique outcome" in a family's history (White & Epston, 1990). Each of these elements is applied to the process of healing (Luckner & Nadler, 1995).

From systems theory's perspective, people are always trying to make sense of their own lives and the things they experience around them. The process of making sense of things involves a never-ending search for and construction of personal meaning. One of the major tenets of systems theory is that in order to learn new information, people must be actively involved in the learning process. Counselors suggest that people do not acquire knowledge from outside information given to them, rather they learn by constructing new meanings from new and old experiences in a context of rich social interaction (Luckner & Nadler, 1995). Several principles of constructivism, adapted from Luckner & Nadler (1995), which are especially applicable to the therapy that will take place in EAP sessions are found in Table 2.2.

Reconstructing the Family Story

In essence, stories become a way of capturing the complexity, specificity, and interconnectedness of an experience and conjoining them into coherent, meaningful, unified themes (Luckner & Nadler, 1995). From a systems theory's perspective, it is intended that people live storied lives; human beings think, perceive, imagine, and make choices according to narrative structure (Luckner & Nadler, 1995). Stories are constructions that give meaning to events and convey a particular sense of experience (Luckner & Nadler, 1995).

The process of transforming experience into story is so much a part of daily existence that people usually are not aware of its operation (Luckner & Nadler, 1995). Rather, they build stories from the information provided by experience, from the inventory of stories or pre-packaged expectations and ways of interpreting supplied by their culture and from those significant individuals that they interact with in their lives.

Table 2.3 Processing Reflections from a System's Perspective

- The goal is to maximize the number of alternative stories and unusual unique outcomes witnessed and give a voice to them. Comments should be generative.
- Be curious about how the family was able to achieve what they did. Describe what you were surprised by in individuals or the family as a whole and wonder what future changes may be.
- Focus on experiences that are judged by the family members to be preferred developments or developments that the family believes might expand their personal story.
- Family members should actively interview one other. They should not merely point out the positives.
- Remain aware of the various histories, narratives, and metaphors that were expressed by the family members and use the language that they used.
- Try to suspend judgment or the urge to figure things out, assess or diagnose others. The goal is to open up space for new discoveries and stories by asking for deep thinking.
- Keep the process short and devoid of jargon.

Systems theory helps people to co-create their new stories as well as help them re-create more positive perspectives of old stories. By helping them become aware of and articulate the narratives they have developed to give meaning to their lives, members are then able to examine and reflect on the themes they are using to organize their lives and to interpret their own actions and the actions of others (Luckner & Nadler, 1995). Shown in Table 2.3 is a list of key components incorporated within therapeutic recreation processing adapted from Luckner & Nadler (1995), which help people construct and retain new self stories. This perspective is relevant in both group and/or individual settings in EAP as well.

Therapist's role

Systems theory's focus of attention will be on the information that is useful, constructive, helpful, and empowering (Luckner & Nadler, 1995). First, the therapist will ask questions about the quality of existence and the freedom of choice that the family's narrative allows. Second, they will pay attention to events and attributes of the experience, not accounted for by the narrative, which can challenge and test the story as told. And, third, the therapist will offer alternative narratives that incorporate the person's life events in a more coherent and powerful narrative (Luckner & Nadler, 1995).

This method is easily adapted to experiences. First, people witness each other in an activity, as they normally would. Second, when the activity is over, the members create their own story about the experience they recently had, possibly responding to some of the observations suggested above in Table 2.3. Third, the people have a conversation among themselves, commenting on what they saw by asking unusual questions to generate some alternative stories. Fourth, the members have a conversation about what they just heard from one other. In effect, the counselors become co-authors with the members in their new story, as the clients will notice a different or unusual strength or resource (Luckner & Nadler, 1995).

Integrating Second-Order Change

Defining a problem in solvable terms is half the battle, according to systems therapists (Haley, 1978). Reframing the truth that the clients bring into treatment can allow the therapist, and then the members, to discover new meanings and new solutions to a previously stuck relational morass (Watson, 1997). First-order change certainly has its place and, in fact, comprises much of daily life and problem solving. Much can be done within the rules of a given situation to make things run more smoothly. However, there comes a time when more of the same will not suffice, and a shift to another level is required in order to devise an adequate solution. This is the challenge of second-order integration: attending not only to the content of the discussion, but also the manner in which the discussion is framed. **Second-order integration** is that which changes not just what one thinks, but also how one thinks. A Systems' therapist will take a person to a different place, and will open up new vistas that have not been visible before. One final contribution of systems theory's perspective for integrative thought is the challenge to examine the difference, or lack thereof, made by a person's ideas (Watson, 1997). Oliver and Miller (1994) summarize systems theory's goal with a metaphor demonstrating the lasting effects of second-order change, "Give me a fish, and I'll eat for a day; teach me to fish, and I'll eat for a lifetime" (p. 154).

Although many theories and approaches to therapy can be utilized in an EAP session, the five theories explored in detail in this chapter summarize the methodology and philosophy behind EAP. The interactions of the horse also reveal these theories in action which make EAP very unique from other traditional uses of the theories. Clearly, an understanding of the theories and benefits can greatly impact an EAP experience for a client.

Topics for Discussion:

1. *Describe how the facilitator might process the session from each of the five theoretical orientations exclusively (for instance, what might a Cognitive-Behavioral therapist focus on in the processing phase of an EAP session)? What might be different with each approach and what might be similar?*

2. *What are the advantages to being knowledgeable about the theoretical orientation of EAP?*

CHAPTER 2

3. *Can a psychodynamic therapist utilize EAP? Explain.*

Chapter Notes

Chapter Notes

3 WHY HORSES?

Objectives:
- **Explore benefits of horses in therapy**
- **Compare horses to other animals**
- **Discuss characteristics of the horse that help clients change**

In this chapter, we will discuss horses as the key to effectiveness for Equine-Assisted Psychotherapy (EAP). For many reasons, horses are the animal of choice in this form of experiential therapy. We will explore in detail factors that contribute to their significant impact in therapy. We will compare horses to other animals also being used in animal-assisted therapies around the world. There are pros and cons to using any animal as a co-therapist. Nevertheless, horses offer so many unique advantages that the risks are outweighed. It is these unique characteristics that help generate healing, growth, and learning for many across the age span.

Advantages of Horses

We are often asked, "Why horses? Why not other animals?" The answer is not easily expressed in words. However, anyone who has spent much time around horses understands a piece of this indescribable mystery. Regarding the portion of their effectiveness that can be put into words, the following can be said: Horses have long been a part of our society and have been "man's help-mate" for generations. Before automobiles, horses were heavily relied upon for transportation, harvesting, and other work related duties. The spiritual and emotional connection and insight one can gain from a horse is ineffable. Their large stature is intimidating yet empowering for clients struggling with a life issue that seems bigger than they are. Horses are honest teachers about relationships, problem solving, wants and needs. Horses represent power and control. Horses are trainable, adaptable, and teachable -- all characteristics which are imperative for survival in today's chaotic and ever-changing society. Horses are much like humans in that they are social animals. Like adolescents, they would rather be with their peers having fun. Often, they seem stubborn and defiant. They offer unconditional friendship and provide immediate and honest feedback. They are sensitive to nonverbal stimulus which provides valuable, visible lessons in terms of nonverbal body language. Horses are large and powerful, which creates a natural opportunity for some to overcome fear, develop confidence, and explore respect. The size and power of the horse are naturally intimidating to many people.

The horse activities provide a visible metaphor for life experiences and relationships. These metaphors are used to teach people valuable tools for success in life. Participants learn about themselves and others through horse activities and then have the opportunity to discuss related feelings, behaviors, and patterns immediately with their treatment team. Most importantly, participants are able to experiment with new behaviors and choose which behavior will enhance their quality of life and relationships (Thomas, 1999).

Animal-assisted therapy actually had its beginnings with therapeutic horseback riding programs in Germany during the 1960s. It was not until the 1980s that the use of animals in therapeutic settings became more popular in the United States (Wright, 1998). Animals used in various visitations and therapy settings can vary – dogs, cats, horses, Capuchin monkeys, and some varieties of birds are used (Clay, 1997). All animals can be very therapeutic and all may have their place and significance in therapy. Nevertheless, horses seem to stand out for several reasons as the animal of choice for many clients.

Comparison to Other Animals

The use of domesticated animals for therapeutic purposes has gained popularity over the last 20 years (Cole & Gawlinski, 1995; Stanley-Hermanns & Miller, 2002). Dr. Sockalingam and his colleagues (2008) thoroughly and concisely summarized the vast benefits of animal-assisted therapy when they reported:

> *Studies show improvements in patients after interacting with animals have emerged from physical health, cardio-vascular status (Anderson et. al, 1992; Friedman et. al, 1984), and areas of bereavement (Akiyama et. al, 1986). Psychological benefits in areas such as depression (Francis et. al, 1985, Siegal, 1990), aggression (Kanamori et. al, 2001), and stress and anxiety (Barker & Dawson, 1998; Beck et*

al., 1986; Davis, 1988; Siegal, 1990) have all been well-documented in the literature. Animals have had an impact on owners' general sense of well-being (Rowan & Beck, 1994), facilitating humor (McMullough, 1981) and reducing loneliness in the elderly poplutaion (McMullough, 1981; Goldmeier, 1986). A five-year longitudinal study demonstrated fewer doctor visits in pet-owners versus non-owners (Headey et al., 2002).

Therapists have discovered that having an animal in the office, whether it be a cat, a dog, or fish in a tank, is relaxing. Animals help soothe agitated feelings. They can be used as a way to make contact with a reserved client or a hesitant child. An animal may serve as a bridge to person-to-person interaction. If a person is paranoid, he or she may have difficulty connecting with you, whereas the animal acts as a go-between (Sneider, 1992).

A study of a twice-weekly animal visitation program in rest homes using experimental and control groups showed a significant change in residents' functioning. Those who received visits experienced statistically significant decreases in depression, anxiety, and confusion (Burke, 1992). Studies also indicated that visitors to nursing homes who were accompanied by an animal drew more positive interactive responses from the residents than those who came without them. The residents who were exposed to pets smiled more, were more alert, and were less physically aggressive. Patients were noticeably more tolerant of others standing near them when an animal was present (Burke, 1992).

There are also significant physiological effects as well. A person's heart rate is lower when he or she sits quietly or reads aloud in the presence of a friendly animal than when doing so alone. The survival rate for heart surgery patients is higher for those who have pets in their homes than for those who don't. Those who own pets tolerate stress better and have lower cholesterol and blood pressure levels (Wolcott, 1993).

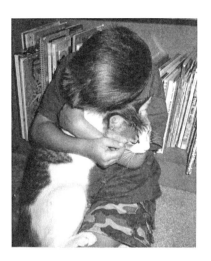

Figure 3.1 One of the benefits of using a cat in therapy is the soothing purr which gives immediate positive and comforting feedback to a client struggling with building positive relationships.

Cats

Cats have been allowed in our environment because they serve a purpose in our society. Cats have co-evolved with humans for centuries. Because this relationship has been one of cohabitation, cats have been allowed to continue their existence primarily independent of humans but tolerant of one another. Due to this fact, they act very independently and are not easily swayed or manipulated for the sake of pleasing others.

In this way, cats tend to be more like people in that they are self-reliant and independent. These characteristics are encouraged in our society but are not always in our best interest, especially when we are in crisis. The cat's innate responses when compared to humans lead to isolation and loneliness in relationships. Cats are very strong willed, sneaky, and are known to have nine lives for a reason. They live life on impulse thinking merely for themselves. Sound familiar? These traits in humans often lead to trouble in relationships. For years, our society has used associations to cats when referring to human relations/actions. Terms such as "cat fight," "cathouse," or "cougar woman," and the list goes on. Well, these are not necessarily the most positive word-pictures.

On the other hand, cats, like other animals, can be very comforting and great companions, when they want to be. Cats have their positive traits that are very therapeutic in the appropriate settings.

However, when considering the modality design, the metaphors to human behavior and problem-solving can only go so far when compared to a cat.

Dogs

Some animals, especially dogs, give unconditional acceptance. They don't care if you're on drugs, inebriated, or HIV positive. When that animal walks up to you, you discover that it wants to connect with you regardless of your circumstances. Dr. Ashok Bedi, a psychiatrist at Milwaukee Psychiatric Hospital, has suggested that animals can fulfill the needs people have to feel valuable and lovable and to sense that they belong and are competent. Animals don't talk back, criticize, or give orders (Wright, 1998).

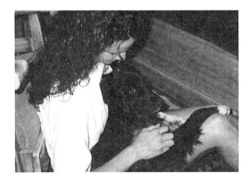

Figure 3.2
Therapy dogs can be very loving and accepting companions which can be very useful in helping a reluctant client open up.

A year long study of nearly 1,000 elderly members of a Los Angeles health maintenance organization discovered that those who owned dogs sought medical care 20% less often than those without pets (Wright, 1998). Dogs have been used for years with the sight impaired. Now, with the hearing impaired, dogs are used to alert their owners to sounds such as a baby's cry, phone, doorbell, alarm clock, or smoke detector (Fraser, 1989). Some dogs have rare abilities to help their owners. For instance, Walton, a Labrador-mix service dog, is a seizure-alert dog, able to warn his owner of impending epileptic attacks before they strike. Once his owner, Emily, has had a seizure, the dog is very protective and won't allow her to exert herself the next day (Christie, 1997).

A study by Allen and Blascoush explored by Clay (1997) showed that dogs were actually a better source of social support than spouses. Two-hundred forty people participated in this stress study, which showed that participants' stress response was highest when spouses were present and lower when only their pets were there. The conclusion was drawn that it's probably because dogs are non-judgmental or perceived that way (Clay, 1997).

Although dogs have many traits similar to that of a horse, dogs are predators -- not prey animals and this difference dramatically changes the way they handle fear. When the overwhelming sense of fear arises for a dog, the natural instinct to attack returns. The domesticated dog of today still expresses his position on the ladder of social studs, just as he did when he lived in the wild state. Dogs, in a large pack, range in order of social status from the most dominant, who is the pack leader, down to the most submissive. Such disputes often erupt into severe fights with possible fatal consequences (Tucker, 1994).

It can be argued that these innate predator traits are also present in humans, as we are predators as well. Therefore, we hold similar responses when responding to fear. This is not always the most helpful response for relationships. Just as with cats, our society has used associations to dogs when referring to these negative human relations/actions. Terms such as "he/she is such a dog" (or female dog—to even be more descriptive), "treats him/her like a dog," and the list goes on. Again, these are not necessarily the most positive word-pictures.

When people are involved, most domesticated dogs, especially therapy dogs, automatically give the human the higher social ranking without the battle. This takes away from many therapeutic opportunities for growth in learning how to earn respect from others. If the client were to have to earn the dog's respect and social order ranking as other dogs do, it could create some safety concerns due to the innate aggressive nature of the natural positioning establishment process in a dog's pack.

As a result of the fact that dogs have been domesticated as companions for man, many of the innate dog traits have been numbed and superseded by the dog's strong desire to please his master. With this occurring, a dog becomes easily manipulated and a people-pleaser. Dogs are bred to give their owners what they want. Furthermore, the good-nature and high socialization of therapy dogs creates an even more agreeable and compliant co-therapist than the everyday dog. All qualities are desirable for emotional and psychological growth within self-esteem, self-worth, and unconditional acceptance; nevertheless, these characteristics limit the client in learning relational skills to survive in the world of complex and ever-changing relationships. The client's opportunity to learn adaptability and flexibility as well as compromise are limited with the dog/client relationship.

Horses

All the animals previously mentioned as being used in animal-assisted therapies are predator animals, except the horse. The word association aspect of what horses represent in our culture are words such as "power," "freedom," and "work-horse." Whereas, the only negative term I could recall is "old nag." So, even the terms we use to associate with horses leave a more positive word-picture for many. Nevertheless, the predator versus prey difference is the most significant difference when discussing possible therapeutic benefits and safety considerations.

A predator animal's nature when fearful or threatened is to attack. Predator animals tend to be more independent and rely less on others when under stress. These characteristics are often present in humans as well. They are frequently the very behaviors that bring a client to therapy – feelings of loneliness and isolation in relationships.

Being a prey animal, horses most often run when they feel threatened, as do most people. People may not always physically run but often emotionally disconnect or run from challenging situations. However, horses find comfort in herds and connect together when under stress. Horses are very accessible and user-friendly. Most people have an interest in and fascination with horses which opens the door for therapy to occur. Horses are accepted by society as a symbol of freedom, power, and control.

Horses are masters at relationships – they naturally find the healthy balance between independence and cohesion with others. Horses desire peace in relationships just as humans do. Horses are able to be more neutral upon first encounter than dogs or cats. This allows the relationships built to be based on present behaviors and responses rather than past expectations and or experiences.

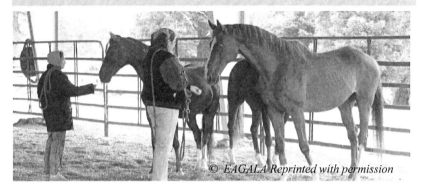

Figure 3.3
Horses provide great opportunities for clients to work on building relationships.

© EAGALA Reprinted with permission

Horses are adaptive to change in social structure and willing to do things out of their natural comfort zone - a skill that people need to learn if they are to have more successful relationships and more meaningful, rewarding lives.

Horses as Teachers

Horses don't lie. They don't separate how they feel from how they act. The expression, "What you see is what you get" could have been coined for a horse. Horses force clients to communicate with the same depth and transparency. Every moment cleints are with them, they're taking measure with the accuracy of a being whose very survival depends on precise readings of its environment. What they need to hear from humans is what many people would like to experience as well. They want people to have a calm, focused assurance. They want others to be consistent. They want people to be both strong and compassionate. Horses need clients to be their best selves. And by being so sensitive to self-doubt and fear, they help clients to find obstacles within themselves and root them out.

The difficult part about working with a horse is not really the horse at all. It's all about knowing who they are, knowing who the horse is, and knowing who they need to be to bring the two together. Horses are experts at non-verbal communication and reading body language to determine authenticity and sincerity. For example, to teach a horse to stop running and be calm, responsive, trusting and brave, the clients must first acquire those qualities in themselves. They can't simply appear confident and in control. Clients must let go of masks, conflicts, and fears and simply be confident and in control.

Everything a client can teach a horse, he/she can teach him/herself. In this process, the client discovers that when a horse sees him/her as relaxed, balanced and centered, so does everyone else. Becoming more horse-like in awareness of the world and how one achieves his/her place in it will make each client a more complete human beings who works and relates well with others, yet knows how to stand his/her ground (Irwin, 2000). What's more, in today's globalized interconnected world, where everyone is affected by the actions of everyone else, what is learned from horses is becoming a necessary stage of human evolution (Irwin & Weber, 2001).

Those who are familiar with horses recognize and understand the power of horses to influence people in incredibly powerful ways. Developing relationships, training, horsemanship instruction, and caring for horses naturally affect the people involved in a positive manner. Working with horses improves work ethic, responsibility, assertiveness, communication, and healthy relationships. Horses naturally provide these benefits.

As discussed earlier, horses are very much like humans in that they are social animals. They have defined roles within their herds. They would rather be with their peers. They have distinct personalities, attitudes, and moods. An approach that seems to work with one horse, does not necessarily work with another. At times, they seem stubborn and defiant. They like to have fun. In other words, horses provide vast opportunities for metaphorical learning. Using metaphors, in discussion or activity, is an effective technique when working with even the most challenging individuals or groups.

Figure 3.4
Horses help clients reflect on their actions, thoughts, & beliefs about life situations.

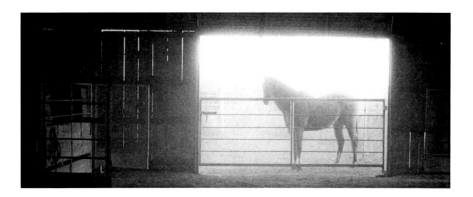

Horses require work, whether in caring for them or working with them. In an era when immediate gratification and the "easy way" are the norm, horses require people to be engaged in physical and mental work to be successful, a valuable characteristic in all aspects of life. Horse activities bring to light the truth in the saying, "Pain of discipline vs. Pain of regret." Horses help people see the reality that either option is painful; the difference is in the long-term and/or big picture.

Most importantly, horses have the ability to mirror exactly what human body language is telling them. Many people will complain, "The horse is stubborn. The horse doesn't like me," but the lesson to be learned is that if they change themselves, the horses respond differently. Horses are honest, which makes them especially powerful messengers.

Topics for Discussion:

1. *Discuss the pros and cons to using horses in therapy? Are there any situations where you feel horses would NOT be appropriate? Explain.*

CHAPTER 3

2. *Explain the differences between a predator vs. prey animal in how it would affect a therapy session and/or client's well being.*

3. *Describe two different life issues that could be targeted in an EAP session? Specifically, what would the horse have to offer in addressing these issues?*

4. *What do you see as the primary benefits to using horses in therapy and the EAP approach? What approach would you take in convincing an agency to fund your EAP program over another animal-assisted therapy?*

Chapter Notes

Chapter Notes

4 BENEFITS OF EQUINE-ASSISTED PSYCHOTHERAPY

Objectives:
- **Identify short-term and long term benefits of Equine-Assisted Psychotherapy**
- **Illustrate impact of EAP through case studies and testimonials**
- **Investigate research in the field**

This chapter will explore the benefits of Equine-Assisted Psychotherapy in depth considering the generalizability and long-term effects of the technique. Being such a new form of therapy, limited quantitative and long-term research has occurred to date. There are mostly qualitative collections of case studies and small sample quantitative data available. In conclusion, this chapter will include available statistics as well as stories of life changing experiences occurring in the EAP arena.

Advantages to Equine-Assisted Psychotherapy

Creates opportunities to practice new skills and to transfer back to life

One of the primary purposes of adventure-based experiences like EAP is to assist people in developing insight and skills that transfer to their lives. Without such positive transfer, EAP would have limited long-term value (Gass, 1993a). Perkins & Salomon (1992) state that "transfer of learning occurs when learning in one context or with one set of materials impacts on performance in another context or with other related materials" (p. 2). The role of the EAP team in facilitating meaningful exchanges of insights, thoughts, feelings, reactions, and the co-constructing of new stories (metaphors) is a delicate and complex one (Luckner & Nadler, 1995). White (1992) summarizes EAP's contributions by saying, "The stories that we enter into with our experience have real effects on our lives. The expression of our experience through these stories shapes or makes up our lives and our relationships" (p. 81). Myers (2009) reinforces that EAP provides metaphorical experiences which facilitate intensive learning. These experiences are more accessible, achievable and memorable for the clients. According to Dyk, Cheung, Pohl, Noriega, and Lindgreen (2013), the follow-up survey results indicated that successful transfer of learning from the horse arena to personal and professional life did occur for subjects.

Involves all aspects of the person to generate change

EAP allows people to build their mental structure on a healthy foundation and also allows reconstruction and restoration of a cracked or crumbling foundation. Healing involves an improvement of the condition of our mind, body, and spirit. When healing is spoken of in EAP, counselors are referring to a process involving physical, emotional, and spiritual dimensions. Healing usually involves all of these dimensions simultaneously. EAP engages the whole person in a natural environment and thus may be an environment ideally suited to holistic healing (Miles, 1993). The healing process uses the resources of the mind, body, spirit, and environment.

Reveals an ability to impact life with decision making and personal responsibility

Another benefit of using horses in therapy is that EAP assists clients in identifying and accessing their own inner capabilities for healing and finding balance in their lives. Through this process, the client becomes increasingly able to assume self-responsibility for life experiences (Howe-Murphy & Murphy, 1987). Clearly, "Change begins with individuals becoming clear and ceasing to act out of misunderstanding and ignorance. This task of moving out of the bondage of individual anger, malice, greed, and self-service is the most formidable challenge of a lifetime" (Pelletier, 1985, p. 31). Shultz (2005) found that those receiving EAP experienced significantly greater amounts of change than the control group in areas such as: intrapersonal distress, interpersonal relationships, social problems, somatic symptoms, and behavioral dysfunction than the control group.

Provides a non-threatening and motivating learning environment

Equine-Assisted Psychotherapy provides clients with many opportunities to explore their true selves in a challenging, accepting, supportive, and conscious environment. The EAP team assists the client in reducing excessive stress; encouraging the development of self-confidence, self-esteem, and a positive mental attitude; and generally creating an environment conducive to well-being and personal expression within relationships. Instead of attempting to "solve" the problems after the damage has been done, EAP can be a more effective answer to problem solving. EAP strengthens relationships and helps people cope with life problems, and as a result, often helps buffer future problems (Wright et al., 1994). This approach does not teach clients how to interact with the horses; rather, it encourages the clients to develop what strategies work best for them (Kelly, 2010).

Empowers clients by giving them a sense of control

Participants experience an increase in self-confidence and a feeling of tranquility. They come to feel that they can deal with whatever challenges the environment may offer them. Miles (1993) suggest that these benefits are in part attributable to the realization that one cannot control a horse. By relinquishing the illusion of control over the animal, participants paradoxically acquire more internal control and can relax and pay more attention to their surroundings and to their inner selves. As a result, EAP enables participants to have confidence in themselves and in their abilities to succeed in the face of frustration -- changing what they can control and identifying what they have no control over. Thus, clients come to feel more and more able to be in control of their lives and to cope with adversity.

Breaks down defense barriers

The structure of an EAP session is unique in that the focus for the client is on activities with horses. This creates a distracter and a focus for the client on something other than the therapist which in part aids the therapist in getting a more authentic picture of the client and issues at hand. The other piece of this formula comes from the horses. In order to have success with the horses, genuine and consistent actions must be conveyed. Horses are masters of non-verbal communication and respond to the most subtle cues. They distinguish quickly between acting and true emotion. With the focus being on accomplishing the horse related task, clients are able to loosen up and relax more quickly and naturally.

Enhances problem-solving skills

Equine-Assisted Psychotherapy requires immediate solutions to problems at hand, which, when practiced on a regular basis nurtures an ability to adapt and the development of problem solving skills. This ability in turn results in a decrease of emotional intensity and fosters learning more effective ways to manage reactions to symptoms and distressing memories or thoughts (Lancia, 2008). The EAP activities are designed to challenge the clients to think outside of their standard means of operation. They are set up as a metaphor for the client's life and/or relationships in some way. A client would not be in therapy if he or she didn't feel "stuck" or at a loss as to what to do with the situation and/or feelings at hand. Therefore, activities mirror the feelings and thoughts that clients most often state such as "can this be done?" or "I have tried everything that usually works but those things aren't working now." With the most obvious solutions not being an option, the client is quickly thrown back into problem-solving mode in order to get results with the horse. The horse's forgiving response to attempts, whether successful or not, helps keep the client going as depicted in Figure 4.1.

Teaches empathy, responsibility, and patience

Everyone has a role in the EAP arena when activities are conducted. It becomes apparent to the clients how their behavior impacts others regarding safety and results. Clients also become aware of whether they consider the horse and others to be involved in activity or if they are so driven toward the goal that they forget about the horses and everyone else. This dynamic becomes very apparent and will create some extra challenges in the arena for clients until they are willing to take a look at their level of consideration for others. Patience is also a skill that is continually challenged and developed in the arena. Anyone who has worked with horses knows that patience is the key to building a solid relationship with your horse. This same concept applies to people as well and is a key component for success within EAP activities.

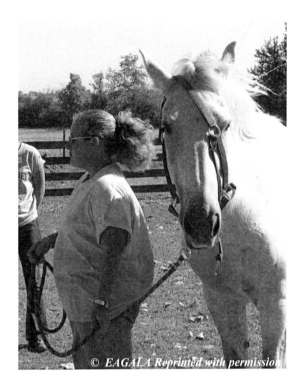

Figure 4.1
Is this haltering attempt right, wrong, or just different? Who or what defines "wrong" for you?

Provides immediate cause and effect situations

Horses operate under the premise of immediate cause and effect because they are constantly taking care of their basic needs. They are simple creatures by the fact that life is very clear to them. Actions they choose now affect the outcomes they get. This concept is a challenging one for many clients but encourages change to occur more rapidly. This natural setting allows consequences to be natural as well. Experiencing the consequences is another benefit to the immediate cause and effect dynamic that occurs in the arena. The client quickly learns that his/her actions will directly influence the response from the horse. Therefore, using the EAP experience therapeutically offers immediate and tangible insights into clients' habitual ways of thinking, behaving, and construing the world (Peel & Richards, 2005).

Builds trust in relationships

EAP activities require much teamwork and communication. This process helps to build trust. The client builds trust in self as well as trust in others. To find success in the activities, the client must establish some degree of trust in the horses as depicted in Figure 4.2. This experience is transferable to other relationships in the client's life. As explained by Dyk, Cheung, Pohl, Noriega, and Lindgreen (2013), horses establish roles within the hierarchical social structure of the herd. Each horse's role is communicated through both subtle and obvious body language. Humans also communicate their roles in relationships by the use of non-verbal cues. Therefore, having horses become the facilitators in learning assists in developing better awareness of these cues which impact teamwork and communication.

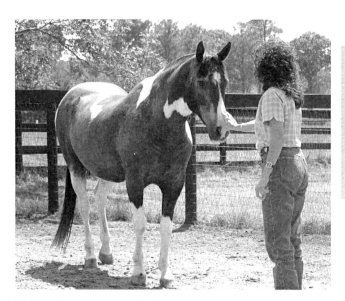

Figure 4.2 Some horses trust you up front; with others, you must earn it. Which type of horse are you?

Stimulates creativity

EAP activities require clients to get creative in their problem-solving, or they will not find success or complete the tasks. Being forced beyond their comfort zone and being faced with a dilemma, the clients must begin to generate new ideas in order to accomplish anything with the horses. Creativity is contagious and one small success leads to more successes. This phenomenon transfers to their lives as well. As soon as the client is able to begin thinking outside the box, s/he will find a whole world of new options that have not yet been explored.

Decreases feelings of hopelessness

As the client begins to realize and experience a core EAP belief that "there is always more than one way to do things," s/he will begin to find new hope that life can get better and the feelings the client is experiencing can now change. According to Shultz (2005), both adolescents and caregivers who participate in EAP experienced statistically significant changes in areas such as depression, anxiety, fearfulness, self-harm and hopelessness. The EAP activities and the horses themselves help the client to see new choices and also experience the unconditional acceptance that is often needed. The horses don't care about the client's rate of success and/or resume; therefore, they are there to care about who the client is rather than basing their value on what the client has done. This experience is refreshing for even the most hopeless clients. The horse is a nonjudgmental, honest friend.

Improves client self-concept

As clients experience success in accomplishing tasks with the horses without help, clients begin to see that they are capable of accomplishing other tasks and goals in life. Through unconditional acceptance, clients begin to believe in their value as a person. Getting a 1200 pound animal to do what is asked is a very empowering experience. The feeling of control over one's actions and decisions helps generate greater self-esteem. This heightened self-esteem reflects back into a client's image of self. In a recent study, Walsh and Blakeney (2013) found that nurses who experienced a one day workshop with the horses "reported being empowered through Equine-Assisted Learning to develop themselves through self-awareness, building confidence, and advanced verbal and nonverbal communication skills" (p. 6).

Increases the client's internal locus of control

Locus of control is the extent to which people perceive outcomes as internally controllable by their own efforts or as externally controlled by chance or outside forces. More specifically, **external locus of control** is the belief that chance or outside forces determine one's fate, while **internal locus of control** is the belief that one controls one's own destiny (Myers, 2010). As clients work with the horses, they will begin to differentiate between what they can control versus that which they have no control. This realization frees clients up to take responsibility for their actions. The clients see how behavior and choices affect the responses of the horses, therefore, affecting the outcome of the activity. Grappling with the options and decisions of how to approach the activity may create some frustration and anxiety for the client at first. Nevertheless, the client feels a greater sense of accomplishment when able to work through it. This shift in locus of control accompanied by the increased self-concept allows clients to move on after therapy and apply the skills learned in session to future events in life.

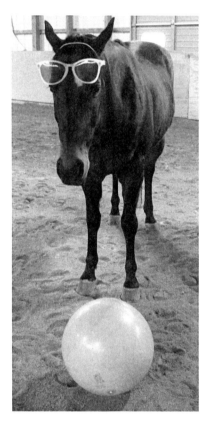

Figure 4.3
This horse is very tolerant of a client's expression of "fun." Sessions give clients the space to be creative without judgment. The horse lets the client know when "enough is enough." Each horse's tolerance threshold is different just as with people.

Captivates and holds attention

Therapists often misconstrue clients' refusal or unwillingness to participate in an activity as being disengaged and uninvolved. This is not true. As long as clients are present and on premises, they are engaged. Studies show that skills such as organization, completion, and concentration improve through EAP and transfer to practical areas of life creating a change in day-to-day functioning for participants (Shultz, 2005).

Working with the horses creates an added advantage of maintaining the client's attention and interest. The horse will often re-involve the client in an activity. Moreover, the therapist must remember that the power of this therapy is the process -- not the content or successful completion of the task. Clients are not able to disengage because everything they do at the barn is part of the EAP process and necessary information.

Conveys lessons on an emotional level

Salovey and Mayers (1990) define **emotional intelligence** (EQ) as "the ability to monitor one's own and others' feelings and emotions, to discriminate among them and to use this information to guide one's thinking and actions" (p.189). The ability to accurately perceive non-verbal signals and body language is closely related to increased emotional intelligence (Cherry, 2013). Recent neurobiological research shows that there are connections in our brains that are involved with both emotion and the way we behave through the use of facial expressions and body language (Gelder, 2006). There is a power within the equine-assisted activities that often generates intense emotions within clients while they are participating. The emotions are very familiar and magnified in the arena. The arena activities and format create a very safe place to explore true emotions increasing emotional intelligence. The horses themselves have a very intimate and sincere affirming presence about them which often encourages clients to be real and vulnerable to their intense emotions within.

Promotes change from dysfunctional patterns to successful ones

All EAP activities require a degree of health and balance to be able to succeed. Some of the qualities necessary to be successful in accomplishing the activities with the horses include: firm but flexible boundaries, trust, consistent and effective communication, teamwork, patience, consideration of others, creativity, and adaptability. All of these qualities come with health and wellness for an individual and/or family. The horse activities require clients to explore and try out new ways of handling difficult situations. According to the study by Shultz (2005), "adolescents are able to recognize and alter maladaptive coping strategies in a concrete way through EAP, it positively affects their psychosocial functioning outside the therapeutic setting. This change is reported by both adolescents and their primary caregivers" (p. 54). Magnelli, Magnelli, and Howard (2009) emphasize that concepts are grasped quickly in the presence of a horse in EAP. This gives clients an opportunity to find success immediately; therefore, success at home is not as difficult because they have the confidence and assurance that they have already been successful.

Stimulates Lasting Impact

The experience of success in completing EAP activities can also enable people to incorporate a new sense of themselves as achievers into their self-structure. From a therapeutic perspective, it could be compared to what Mearns and Cooper (2005) refer to as "touch stones." The therapeutic power of these experiences of change is enhanced by the fact that they are highly distinctive and memorable. A client may make a change in his/her perception of him/herself in a conversation with a therapist and forget what was said as soon as he/she leaves. Clients rarely forget what it was like to catch and halter the massive horse that reminded them of their biggest fear because the physiological effects of endorphin and adrenaline release enhance the impact of the success (Peel and Richards, 2005). The collective aspects of the EAP experience, therefore, provide a context in which clients explore their constructs, behaviors and general approach to life in a direct way. In short, the psychological and physical demands are often so different and more intense than those experienced in everyday life, that they offer long-term psychological benefits (Peel & Richards, 2005; Voight et. al, 2003).

Figure 4.4   Promoting Change

"All of life's accomplishments start with observation." Randy Mandrell, Director of Equine Services, Refuge Services

Increases Awareness of the Present

Horses are very large animals and working with them requires one to become present and aware – much like the horses themselves. A recent pilot study by Walsh and Blakeney (2013) suggests that working with horses increases subjects' abilities to become present. Because horses give feedback on every action made and every emotion held, working with them forces people to engage in first, second, and third level feedback or "action inquiry" (Torbert, 2004). According to Torbert

(1972), **action inquiry** is the process of questioning in relationship with action. He states that "experiential learning involves becoming aware of the qualities, patterns and consequences of one's own experience as one experiences it" (p 7). Clinician Mark Rashid's philosophy of horse training holds true to life as well, which states to find awareness, one must soften his/her body and senses in order to see, hear, and feel what is going on in the moment (Anderson, 2007, p. 18). By increasing awareness about the comfort level of the horse, and getting honest, in-the-moment feedback from them, one can choose to act in ways that make collaboration happen easily and more frequently (Dyk, Cheung, Pohl, Noriega, & Lindgreen, 2013). In a recent study, Walsh and Blakeney (2013) concluded that "Equine-Assisted Learning can be a meaningful venue for self-discovery in their ability to be present." (p. 6).

Research

Equine-Assisted Psychotherapy is a dawning discipline in a rapidly changing field. Due to the newness of the technique, little quantitative data has been reported or analyzed over the long term. Nevertheless, from the case studies and personal testimonies over the years, EAP is showing itself to be highly effective in both its immediate and long-term results.

Based on what we know about experiential learning, it has been estimated that while we remember only 20% of what we hear and 50% of what we see, we retain fully 80% of what we do. As a result, there is great momentum for understanding the nature and power of experiential education and how it can make use of the way the human nervous system is wired to learn (Smolowe, Butler, Murray, 1999). These activity-based experiences like EAP have greater sticking power than traditional-style trainings where participants sit and receive information via lecture, overhead and video.

Overall, the benefits to the participants are immediate and are measurable. Results show attainment of basic skills, competency, and maturity in thinking. Clients also report an increase in productive and positive relations with peers, teachers, parents, co-workers, and other individuals. As a result of learned skills and confidence, participants increase the amount of involvement in school, work, and community activities while using creativity in a positive manner. For example, Tetreault (2006) found that behavior management skills increased on average by 34% through group EAP, as well as a 22% increase in communication and social skills among those participating. In addition, participants report a decrease in the amount of eating disordered behavior, depression, anxiety, violent outbursts, drug/alcohol problems, and other anti-social behaviors upon completion (Shultz, 2005).

Most research focuses on what problems exist and how often they occur rather than on what contributing factors occurred at the onset of the problem at hand. Researchers have largely failed to examine factors that help people develop resilience to the stresses of life and relationships. One area of emphasis in EAP is the examination of how encountering and overcoming problems constitutes a resource that contributes to growth in the client and strengthens their relationships (Wright et al., 1994). In sum, EAP's goals include improving stress management skills, building emotional strengths, and enhancing communication skills. EAP explores ways to help people effectively balance cohesion and adaptability to mesh with the needs of others.

Figure 4.5
The most subtle change can be very positive and insightful even in the middle of a complex EAP activity.

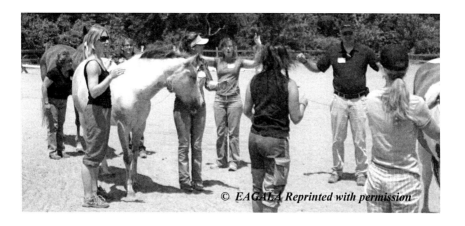

© *EAGALA Reprinted with permission*

A study by Schultz, Remick-Barlow, and Robbins (2007) indicated Equine-Assisted Psychotherapy is effective in improving overall functioning of children who have been diagnosed with adjustment disorder, mood disorders, PTSD, ADHD and disruptive disorder. The study reveals that after an 18-month period of time in EAP all children showed improvement in Children's Global Assessment of Functioning (GAF) scores, and that there was a statistically significant correlation between the percentage improvement in GAF and the number of sessions given in that timeframe (average number of sessions being 19). This study also revealed that the younger children as well as children with a history of intra-family violence and substance abuse showed the greatest improvement in GAF scores (Schultz et. al, 2007).

Klontz, Bivens, Leinart, and Klontz (2007) found that after 28 hours of Equine Assisted Psychotherapy the study participants showed significant and stable reductions in overall psychological distress and enhancements in psychological well-being. The participants reported fewer psychological symptoms and reductions in the intensity of the psychological distress, such as: (1) more oriented in the present; (2) better able to live more fully in the here-and-now; (3) less burdened by regrets, guilt, and resentments; (4) less focused on fears related to the future; (5) more independent; and (6) more self-support. These results remained significant at the six-month follow up.

Trotter, Chandler, Goodwin-Bond and Casey (2008) compare equine-assisted counseling (EAP) to classroom-based counseling. The study indicated that EAP made statistically significant improvements in 17 behavior areas whereas the classroom therapy showed statistically significant improvement in 5 areas. This research found EAP to be effective with at-risk children and adolescents. In addition EAP treatment was determined to be superior to classroom counseling (Trotter, Chandler, Goodwin-Bond & Casey, 2008).

More specifically, in the study children and adolescents who received EAP performed more than three fourths of a standard deviation better than those who received classroom counseling. Improvements on social stress and self-esteem scales indicates that EAP participants' self-satisfaction improved, sense of identity increased, and level of ego strength improved to appropriate levels. It also indicated that hyperactivity reduced significantly. Those receiving EAP demonstrated a noticeable increase in their ability to focus, stay on task, and no longer be overactive. Also, a reduction in verbal and physical aggression behavior was demonstrated by those participating in EAP. A final outcome indicated the reduction in conduct problems such as cheating, lying, stealing, alcohol/drug use, and social deviant and disruptive behavior (Trotter, Chandler, Goodwin-Bond & Casey, 2008).

Trotter, Chandler, Goodwin-Bond, and Casey (2008) conclude, "These results offer validation that EAP is a viable treatment for children and adolescents at risk for social and academic failure. The effect of EAP on internalizing problems as reported by the participants and their parents is particularly promising because it denotes a noticeable increase in participants' ability to internally cope with their problems and seem less lonely, less nervous, and less anxious" (p. 280).

A final study demonstrating the long-term effectiveness of Equine-Assisted Psychotherapy also compares EAP to other forms of intensive therapy. The outcomes are significant and show lasting impact (Mann, 1998). Mann (1998) reports that comparative costs for six months of treatment in the respective programs are as follows: Journey Home EAP program at $3,200, Boot Camp at $5,400 and, inpatient treatment at $27,000. No statistics were available regarding the effectiveness of the inpatient programs.

A Las Vegas, New Mexico EAP program called "Ride to Pride," is the sister program of Journey Home. The Ride to Pride EAP program has demonstrated a 53% success rate with juvenile offenders admitted; 95% of them have maintained these (same targets as this study) targets for a year past graduation (Mann, 1998).

Mann (1998) concluded from his study that the combination of equine involvement and psychotherapy can create dramatic increases in the percentage of juvenile clients who respond favorably to treatment. The increased cost associated with the use of horses is offset significantly by the increase in successful outcomes. The comparative costs of EAP and inpatient treatment indicate tremendous savings by using this innovative method of intensive outpatient treatment.

This research is important when considering the long-term success of programs and therapy. It is imperative that those providing EAP gather more information to support such an impressive form of therapy. Clearly, more quantitative research needs to be conducted in this field to further demonstrate the effectiveness and long-term outcomes of this approach.

Case studies

Personally, I have many success stories demonstrating the benefits of Equine-Assisted Psychotherapy. The more I practice EAP, the less I do traditional therapy. I see results much more quickly and observe clients better retaining what they are learning. Also, I notice clients are applying these new skills in their lives. A few case studies in particular demonstrate this transformation. All names and identifying information have been changed to protect the privacy of the clients.

Amy's Story

Amy was a young professional in the mental health field. She came to a treatment center because she was struggling with an eating disorder, anorexia. When she first arrived, she was so underweight that she had to be put on a liquid diet before her body would even accept food. She continually battled with the thoughts that she was fat and striving for perfection. Conventional therapy was challenging in the beginning because of her knowledge of therapy. She knew what to say and also knew what she should be doing. She was just unable to bypass her strong emotions and thoughts that were leading her to destruction. She was caught in a vicious cycle. The horses were something Amy had never experienced before in a therapy setting. It was challenging, yet very rewarding for her. During her three months stay at the residential program, she worked with the horses on a daily basis. The horses brought her insight into her physical, emotional, relational, and spiritual existence. Over the three months, I began to see Amy's spirit come alive again as she regained control over herself and over her eating disorder. The horses helped her learn to discern what she had control over versus what she did not. The horses taught her new problem-solving skills and gave her renewed confidence in herself. Amy's words, when asked what she gained from her EAP experience, were as follows:

> *"My experience in EAP and with the horses in general was probably the most valuable part of my recovery. Not only did I overcome an eating disorder, but I also learned more about myself mentally, physically, and spiritually. In fact, I am now pursuing my Master's degree in social work and hope to one day be an EAP specialist myself!"*

When Amy was leaving residential treatment after her three months of recovery, she stated:

> *"The horses have shown me that there is such a thing as unconditional forgiveness, there is such a thing as unconditional love, and that the capability exists to love without reservation or judgment. No matter what I may have done to the horse the day before (i.e. forcing him to do something that he didn't want to do, making him work extra hard, etc.), I could come out to the pen the next day, and that same horse nuzzled up to me again. EAP itself brought many truths to light for me. They were always present in the horses; I just didn't see them until EAP brought them out."*

It was apparent that EAP taught Amy patience, contentment, and joy in the moment. She had to have these things when she was with the horses because they didn't respond if she wasn't patient with them and "fully present" – meaning continuously aware of her thoughts, actions, and surroundings. In everyday life, she discovered this realization that she needed to be "fully present." Her eating disorder was taking away her life, so that while her body was there (what little was left of it), her spirit was lost. In order to be who she wanted to be, she had to discover how to be "fully present" in each and every day. In EAP, if her body was there and her mind was not, not only did she miss important opportunities, she also exposed herself to the risk of injury. In her every day life, she realized that if she was not "fully present," she risked losing out on important points and opportunities, as well as exposing herself to injury or danger.

Amy has moved on to continue her education as a social worker and after two years, she is married and doing well. She is no longer battling an eating disorder. She has progressed professionally as well as relationally.

Sally's Story

Sally got out of her parent's car with a sour look on her face. She would not make eye contact or interact with the other teenagers that were there for group therapy. She had been coming for about three weeks, yet very little change had occurred in behavior. She was suffering with depression and suicidal thoughts from time to time. She did like the horses and being with them kept her coming back. This week, we were doing an activity called "Extended Appendages." In the activity, the group was divided into teams of three. The person in the middle was the brain and the two on either sides of the brain were the "appendages," or arms. The brain's job was to explain to the arms how to saddle the horse. The brain could not use her own arms, while the arms couldn't think for themselves. The trio locked arms and began. Sally's group was a diverse one. The brain was tall and athletic; the left arm was small and intimidated, and Sally. Sally was dressed in all black and never made eye contact with her group. The group began. The brain began giving instruction to the arms about how to saddle the horse. The saddle was very awkward and heavy. The small client and Sally were having a very difficult time lifting the saddle. Sally let go of the saddle and sat down on the ground. She stated, "I quit." The two others left looked at me as if to say, "How are we supposed to get this done now?" My immediate thoughts were, "Oh great. Now they can't finish. Someone else will have to join their team or they will just have to watch the others." Then, I remembered that the process is what is important in this activity, not the outcome. With this in mind, I stated to the two remaining clients staring in state of concern, "Do your best. It looks like you lost an arm here but you must go on." They worked so hard but were unable to get the saddle up because the small arm was the only one able to lift. The brain asked Sally many times to please help but she refused. She sat at the foot of the horse the entire activity and watched in amazement as the two others struggled without her. She began to cry.

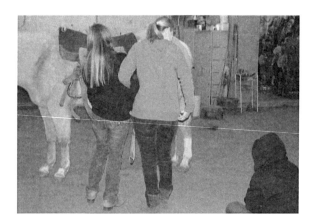

Figure 4.6
Many times situations are not as they appear. The facilitator must not assume they know what experience clients are having in an activity.

After the activity was through, we began to process what everyone got from this activity. Many significant lessons were revealed, but Sally's lesson seemed to be the most profound of all. Just when we thought she had quit, she actually was experiencing a breakthrough. After hearing the two boys again verbalize how difficult it was to work on the task without Sally's help, Sally stated, "I learned that others need my help more than I think sometimes. If I don't do my part, they will have a hard time without me. When I help others it feels really good. I never knew that I really was important to anyone."

Sally was never the same after this activity; she began interacting with the other teenagers in the group and making eye contact when talking to the group. Her depression began to lift and thoughts of suicide disappeared.

This experience reminded me, once again, to be open to whatever happens in an EAP session and to not get so focused on my agenda that I am unable to allow the process to do its part. Remember, even when clients appears disengaged or uninvolved, they may possibly be getting exactly what they need from the session.

Figure 4.7
EAP is looking at the experience from a different perspective.

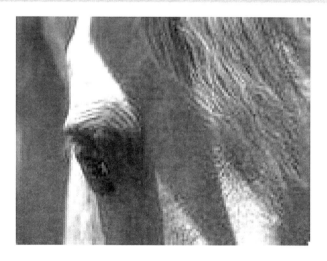

CHAPTER 4

Beth's Story

  While conducting a workshop for other professionals about EAP, I met Beth. Beth was attending the workshop with her mother. I noticed Beth had her small dog with her at all times. She was very quiet and stuck closely with her mom. This was a very large training, so I didn't get a chance to visit much with Beth or her mother except to learn that Beth was with her because she had some trauma issues and refused to stay at home. Her mom said she would leave the training if it was an issue for Beth to be with her. Not seeing any harm in her attendance, I allowed her to participate.

  On the third day of the training, Beth volunteered for an activity. She also wanted her mom to volunteer with her. Her mom agreed. Before the activity started, the volunteers had to choose a consequence that they all would be subject to if anyone broke a rule. Beth spoke up and suggested rolling in horse manure, "poop." The audience gasped. With many other suggestions coming from the audience, I questioned the volunteers numerous times about their options. The more the audience was appalled with the "poop" idea, the more the volunteers were certain that "poop" was going to be their consequence.

  So with their adamancy on this consequence and knowing what I did about Beth's past, I chose to accept their consequence and allow them to proceed. I knew that the fact that Beth was up in front of this large group and speaking up was probably very significant for her. The volunteers proceeded with the activity. Being a demonstration, we only had about 15 minutes for the volunteers to work on the activity; nevertheless, within that small amount of time, they had to roll in "poop" three times. Beth was the leader, as she led the volunteers to the smallest, driest pile and sat down to roll. She laughed the entire time. The rest of the volunteers followed. The audience continued to be aghast that this was being tolerated.

  After the time was up, we began to process. Once again, the audience's focus went directly back to the consequence. The volunteers stated that the consequence was no big deal to them. Beth stated that it would have been more humiliating to sing to the audience than to roll in the "poop" because she has to clean horse stalls every day. During the interrogation from the audience, I noticed the horse move up blocking Beth's view of the audience. Beth began to weep quietly. The audience couldn't see this occurring. She quickly regained her composure before the audience noticed as I began to wrap up questioning and allowed the volunteers to sit down.

This situation was a very controversial one. Many professionals had issues that the treatment team allowed the volunteers to roll in horse manure. That was the audience's main issue but NOT an issue for the volunteers. When the treatment team's agendas and/or beliefs begin to be challenged, it is imperative to be able to sit those aside long enough to observe without judgment what is occurring in the arena. Once observation has occurred, then the treatment team must make a decision as to what to do with the information they have just been given.

Many pivotal points within EAP are a judgment call. A question I would encourage the treatment team to ask themselves when faced with such issues, "Am I projecting my personal issues, judgments, and/or agendas on the client?" Countertransference, bringing personal issues into the therapy session, can interfere in allowing the clients to gain what is needed for their healing. However, the tipping point here is how the treatment team handles what happens. Everything that happens in the arena is part of the process. It is all potential metaphors that can assist the client in relating the arena experience to life. The most negative impact occurs when the treatment team's countertransference regarding any situation becomes the focus over the client's experience. This concept and process will be discussed further in Chapters 14 and 17.

Figure 4.8
Allowing the clients to tell their stories and trusting the process are key components to the success of this approach in therapy. By keeping our own agendas and interpretations out of the way, we are able to take a glimpse into the life of our client for that moment.

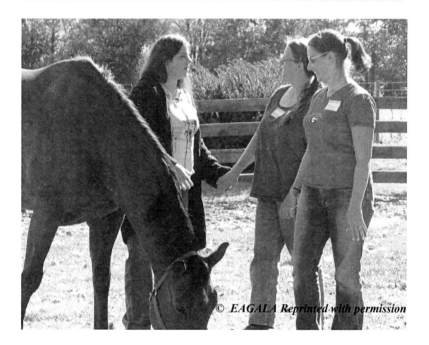

© *EAGALA Reprinted with permission*

In Beth's session, the benefits from making the judgment call to allow the volunteers to follow through with the consequence they chose resulted in far more than I could have ever planned. After the workshop, I received a note from the mom stating that in 15 minutes of EAP the following resulted as shared in Figure 4.9:

Figure 4.9 Beth's Letter

    Thank you for allowing Beth to attend with me. It wasn't planned. Beth had a breakdown at the thought of me leaving her with friends or family and so I made a last minute decision to bring her with me and leave for home if she became disruptive. I hadn't planned on Beth participating in the role playing either, but since she asked to participate and will not normally do anything where she might be noticed, I went with the flow and gave her the okay.

    Beth has been a kid in crisis for the past 6 years. Beth has spent the last 6 years running away from her feelings concerning the eighteen wheeler wreck and being trapped. Three long psych. hospital stays, a trauma center stay, 6 psychologists, 6 years of talk therapy, EMDR therapy, buckets full of psychotropic medications, and everything else under the sun would not encourage Beth to discuss her feelings and fears. Since the wreck, Beth has shut down, refused to talk, falls asleep and/or have meltdowns, developed schizophrenic episodes, dissociative episodes, suicidal attempts and ideation, irrational fears/phobia, incessant elephant man type of hives, amongst many other symptoms. Shadow (her dog) and her ponies have been the only things that keep her going.

    Beth went from being a loving, confident, happy, driven, and two years ahead in school child to a child who couldn't get past fifth grade, violent to strangers/animals, and a reclusive ticking time bomb. Beth has been in Special Ed. for the past four years, is currently homebound from school because she kept hiding under desks and frightening the other children and so much more. We were about a week away from putting Beth back in psych. hospital.

    On the way home from the seminar on Friday night, Beth started telling young Hannah and me that the seminar and role playing was fun and she enjoyed participating.

    She started talking about Thursday's exercise. She said she really enjoyed the temptation alley and consequences game. When it came to discussing the exercise part she said the audience's glares and whispers felt like the eighteen wheeler aiming at us and ready to hurt. Mikey (the horse) put himself between the danger and her and kept her safe.

    She said that it was like the crash. She was trapped and her Mom was unconscious. People (the other volunteer & facilitators) were trying to get her door open to get her out but couldn't pry it open (other volunteer were not able to get the horse to move & facilitators were not able to get the audience to stop interrupting). She said that when the horse walked forward toward her on his own and put himself between her and the audience, it was like when her Mom (me) came to and ran round and pulled the door off, grabbed her out of the truck and ran away from the road with her to safety.

CHAPTER 4

> *She said that her fear was that she thought no one could love her like her Mom, and she was scared of loosing me. She said the horse seemed to understand and put himself in front of the "eighteen wheeler" audience and sheltered her from danger. She said she cried because she realized that she was loved by lots of people and although her Mom (me) loves her the most, others do too, even the horse, who hardly knew her.*
>
> *I asked Beth if she just remembered this (I was knocked out so have no recollections of the wreck or pulling the door off and this was the first time I had ever heard about the door being pulled off) and she said, "no, it was a video running in her head all the time." I asked her why she hadn't told me about this part of the accident before now and she said, "it was too scary to talk about." Beth talked and talked all the way home.*
>
> *She has been a happy kid since being home and no emotional damage seems to have incurred from the "poop" consequence. Beth's psychologist, psychiatrist, teachers, doctors etc. are very excited about Beth's willingness to discuss her feelings and want to learn more about the EAP process and quickly piggy-back on what happened at the training and incorporate this into Beth's therapy. They said Thursday's exercise was Divine intervention and made an enormous psychological break-through with Beth.*
>
> *So in a long thank you, we received more than any one will ever know from the course. The experience on Thursday was placed there for Beth's healing. We were blessed and thank everyone for their participation in this breakthrough.*
>
> *Lots of love, participating mom*
> (anonymous participant, October 10, 2005).

Follow-up on Beth's story. Two to three years later, I came in contact with Beth's mom again at another EAP function. She asked me if I noticed anything different about her? Before I could even respond, she blurted out "Beth isn't with me! She's at school." At that point, she was beaming from ear to ear and gave me a hug. She reported that Beth was doing great. She was back in mainstreamed classes in public school. She was participating in extracurricular activities. She reported that she is smiling and acting like a "typical teenager." She stated that she is continuing with traditional therapy one day per week working on "normal teenager issues rather than the trauma work." She said once again, "thank you for that break through."

Insights from Other Professionals

Professionals around the world speak to the benefits they see with Equine-Assisted Psychotherapy. The personal stories emphasize the impact of the work with more detail than the quantitative statistics are able to measure. Research is limited in its ability to report depth and impact of change when it comes to human awareness, personal growth, and quality of life in this work.

With over 20 years of mental health practice in a residential setting with psychologically unstable children and adolescents, Alspaugh (personal communications, September 29, 2011) frequently turns to EAP as a diagnostic tool. She shares that "what might take you ten sessions in traditional therapy to determine what's going on [with the client], EAP can have done in five." She states that the honesty of the horses is invaluable in therapy. She appreciates the solution-focused model and the fact that a treatment plan can be identified and implemented in a "reasonably quick timeframe" (Alspaugh, 2011).

Zimmerman (2010) describes EAP by saying, "To partner with horses and give someone an opportunity to strengthen their life can be very humbling. Equine assisted learning is very powerful work when people are given the choice of learning by doing (p. 33)." Boyce & Robertson (2008) say that they have no doubts that the horse-client interaction is a powerful one. They have found that clients are not only receptive to EAP but that they "show great initiative and creativity" when they are allowed to develop and create the course of their sessions.

As a professional facilitator for executive training and development, Ron Prince had the opportunity to observe equine-assisted learning and incorporate the processing into his corporate training. Prince (2009) states, "I was amazed at the incredible insights gained throughout the experience. While giving us plenty of fodder for the classroom learning portion of the agenda, I was equally impressed with the metaphors the setting provided for the concept of collaboration (p. 32)."

In 2004, Brady worked with families and children in traditional counseling settings as well as in the EAP arena. She is a believer in pet-therapy as well but concludes that the horses have their unique place in therapy and provide some unique advantages that other therapies cannot provide. Through EAP, she has seen the horses reflect the emotional state and struggles people are having so individually. She has continually experienced the unique way each horse connects with each person so specifically, interested and invested in loving each person where they are and for who they are. Using the horses through EAP teaches clients about joy and laughter and how to laugh at humorous experiences in their lives. She concludes by saying, "EAP allows goodness, love, and joy to come through even under distressing circumstances." (personal communications, June 3, 2004).

Brady shared a story about a client that was very angry and did not want to talk to anyone or deal with anyone. So most of the other clients and staff left her alone. They were unable to break through the wall of resistance. However, one of the horses kept prodding at her, nipping her jacket and arm, and nuzzling into her face with his nose. She walked away, but her horse followed. The horse would not let her resistance throw him off, and soon she was laughing because a 1500 pound animal was following her like a puppy. With the populations Brady has dealt with using EAP, this is a wall that can be very hard to break though, but is so necessary for recovery. "Equine-assisted psychotherapy is a spiritual experience," states K. Brady (personal communications, June 3, 2004).

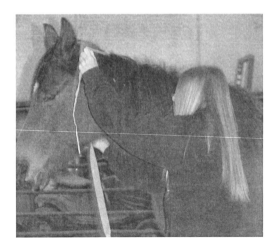

Figure 4.10
The process of healing looks very different for each client.

Brady (2004) goes on to share,

> *God evidences Himself through the horses in EAP. It is a very difficult experience to put into words, just like most experiences with God. You cannot see with your eyes always, what you experience with your heart in the midst of an EAP session. However, I have witnessed even the most spiritually resistant people open their mind and heart in a moment of wonder and awe and begin to really consider that God may exist and love them as a result of experiencing the horses' interaction with them in EAP. I believe that God speaks through each of us to carry His message on earth to others, and I also believe He has equipped animals to do the same. Often, the animals are even more effective than people because they do not bring up the defenses that people do in a hurting heart. So, it's as if God uses the tenderness and unconditional love of the animals to sneak in the back door of a wounded soul. I know that God's truest desire is to love us and for us to feel loved by Him, so that we will desire to obey Him and bring glory to His kingdom with our lives. God has once again, so creatively found another way to express His love and character to his wounded ones (and not-so-wounded ones too) through the use of horses in EAP. I see EAP as one of His gifts to us to help us heal and become more like Him.*

Steve Eller (personal communications, October 1, 2011), an EAP practitioner and University Professor, sums it up best when he concluded that EAP is an observational approach to therapy with a social learning basis providing immediate feedback from the horse to the client. This multifaceted detail about the client gives the facilitators so much to work with. As a result, clients are able to better see the choices and actions they are taking and how those impact the life they are experiencing. This awareness leads to change.

Client Testimonials

Many clients have incorporated Equine-Assisted Psychotherapy into their path to recovery or wellness. In my years as a practitioner, EAP has received much more client feedback than traditional therapy has. I have received numerous thank you notes and phone calls from EAP clients. Some of the comments are as follows:

CHAPTER 4

> "I learned that fear does not help me when I saw Cody (a therapy horse). What I learned about fear was the more fear you have inside of you, it takes a long time to trust someone. I looked at Cody and saw fear. I have had a time like that the first time I came, it was hard for me not to cry or anything due to my fear of the horses. I was not giving the horse a chance. I did not try. That was fear. I now know that my fear can affect my relationships with other people. That's what also helped me. I hope we can all get rid of our fears by the end of the 8 weeks."
>
> Client, age 14

> "I am not hopeless. I can change me even when I can't change what happens to me."
>
> Client, age 14

> "Be as nice as you can, but as firm as necessary. When you're firm, don't get mean or mad. When you're nice, don't act like a wimp. Lightfoot (the horse) taught me that."
>
> Client, age 14

> "Horses taught me how to stand up for myself and to speak up when I don't like something. I have options!"
>
> Client, age 15

> "Don't wait around for things to just happen. You have to not follow the crowd and do your own thing."
>
> Client, age 16

> "I want to thank you so much for all your advice and encouragement over the past few months. I really looked forward every week to our visit. You really brought me through some tough times and did so in a loving environment. I also am thankful that you suggested the horse therapy. I can't even begin to tell you what a blessing that has been for me. I have learned so much about myself and relationships. The horse therapy was far beyond my greatest expectation."
>
> Client, age 21

In some ways, metaphors are the most important protectors of people. When all else fails, there are always memories and stories. They can transcend time and distance, poverty and ill health. These metaphors of food, places, trips, beloved objects and beloved people become the connecting tissue in relationships. They give people's lives a context and meaning, a history and philosophy (White, 1992). EAP is helping clients build positive metaphors and stories to refer to and find hope in.

Topics for Discussion:

1. What do you see as the top five benefits of Equine-Assisted Psychotherapy? Discuss.

2. Many of the benefits listed are also benefits of other experiential therapies. What do you see as the benefits that set EAP apart from other experiential therapies? Explain.

3. What are the disadvantages (if any) for Equine-Assisted Psychotherapy having limited research backing? Discuss.

Chapter Notes

Chapter Notes

Treatment Team

5 THE ROLE OF THE MENTAL HEALTH PROFESSIONAL

Objectives:
- **Identify qualifications for EAP Mental Health Professionals**
- **Explore tasks and skills needed as a professional**
- **Analyze responsibilities of the Mental Health Professional**
- **Evaluate therapist's role in planning and facilitating sessions**

This chapter will look at the importance of the mental health professionals' role in an EAP session. We will discuss the qualifications, ethical considerations, skills and responsibilities, as well as facilitation considerations that a mental health professional must consider when participating as part of an EAP treatment team. Hunter, Luna, Maglio, & Mandrell (2010) summarize the importance of the mental health professional's role in the Equine-Assisted Psychotherapy team in the following way:

> *It is important to be deliberate in your choice of team members. Just as it is important and professional to have people trained in first aid present to handle a physical emergency, it is equally professional and important to have present someone trained in handling emotional "emergencies...." Having a MHP present at all times is an important standard for the professionalism, quality and accountability of services being provided.*

Therefore, in this chapter we will emphasize the fact that a licensed, mental health practitioner is imperative for any Equine-Assisted "Psychotherapy" session to even take place. Clearly, without the therapist, treatment cannot be considered psychotherapy.

Tasks and Skills Needed

Licensing

Equine-Assisted Psychotherapy mental health professionals have many licensing and ethical considerations to act in accordance with, just as all mental health professionals must consider in practice. Specifically, EAP mental health professionals need to have a college-level degree and training in a mental health field, such as social work, psychology, marriage and family therapy, or others that include mental health in its scope of practice. These professionals must counsel within their scope of practice and follow state laws and regulations regarding mental health practice. EAP mental health professionals should operate under a governing board that can hold them accountable (or under professional supervision by a supervisor that is held accountable by a governing board), i.e. a board that can revoke registration, certification, or licensure for ethical or scope of practice violations related to mental health practice (Kersten & Thomas, 2004).

Ethical Considerations

It is the ethical obligation of the EAP mental health professional to operate in accordance to his/her licensing code of ethics, as well as ensure that all members of their treatment team are in accordance and familiar with the therapist's ethical duties. The EAP mental health professionals should refer to the appropriate licensing board in their state to see what these ethical standards are for them and their EAP team. An example of an additional ethical framework is outlined by the international Equine Assisted Growth and Learning Association, EAGALA, an EAP certifying organization.

Building on the work of others, Corey, Corey and Callanan (1998; 2011) describe six basic moral principles that form the foundation of functioning at the highest ethical level as a professional: autonomy, nonmaleficence, beneficence, justice, fidelity, and veracity. Applying each of these principles is not as easy as it may appear due to the complexity of treatment issues and cultural diversity. Nevertheless, they provide a nice overview for mental health professionals to refresh their memory as to the ethical areas of concern as well as provide a springboard for mental health professionals to use when discussing ethical obligations with their horse professionals. In Table 5.1, these six basic moral principles defined by Corey, Corey and Callanan (1998; 2011) are described:

Table 5.1 Six Moral Principles

> ➢ *Autonomy* refers to the promotion of self-determination, or the freedom of clients to choose their own decisions.
> ➢ *Nonmaleficence* means avoiding doing harm, which includes refraining from actions that risk hurting clients, either intentionally or unintentionally.
> ➢ *Beneficence* refers to promoting good for others.
> ➢ *Justice,* or fairness, means providing equal treatment to all people.
> ➢ *Fidelity* means that professionals make honest promises and honor their commitments to those they serve.
> ➢ *Veracity* means truthfulness, including informed consent.

Professional codes of ethics are indeed essential for ethical practice, but merely knowing these codes is not enough. The challenge comes with learning how to think critically and knowing ways to apply general ethical principles to particular situations. An important part of this openness is a willingness of the therapist to focus on him/herself as a person and as a professional as well as on the questions that are more obviously related to the clients (Corey et. al, 1998).

Applying an EAP World View

The therapist in this EAP team not only needs to be skilled in the traditional aspects of counseling to promote effective therapy but also must be someone who is able to think abstractly and able to stand back without intervening and allow the process to have the power. As well, this therapist must be able to work well in a team or with a co-facilitator. As a therapist, the two most difficult skills to master are: (1) having the ability to allow the clients to struggle and work through challenges at their pace and (2) seeing everything that takes place from the time they arrive to the time they leave as therapy and metaphorical for life.

The ability to allow clients to work through an activity at their own pace without intervening or rescuing is very challenging for many EAP professionals. In EAP, the struggles tend to be magnified and very obvious to someone from the outside looking in to see. This challenge seems to be intensified by the fact that the therapist is actually seeing what the clients are doing before your eyes rather than just talking about it. Many times, a solution may seem quite obvious and the client may be begging for answers; nevertheless, to truly maximize this experience and increase the generalizability of the experience, the therapist must allow the client to find an answer for themselves.

Secondly, continuous thinking in pictures or metaphors is a skill that grows with practice. The more the therapist works to think in pictures, the easier and quicker it becomes. Some people are wired to think more so in pictures (visual learners) and this skill may be a bit easier for them. Nevertheless, it is a skill that improves with practice. Within this, it is important for the therapist to begin training the client to think in metaphors as well. This teaching component is very valuable to the client and helpful in aiding the client in finding life lessons within all activities and situations.

Planning and Facilitating Individual Sessions

Psychotherapy requires an explicit contract between client and counselor that spells out expectations, provides focus for the counseling session, and increases client involvement (Young, 1992). Just as in traditional therapy, the initial paperwork and intake information needs to be obtained and covered to ensure the client is informed. This intake paperwork will need to include any additional paperwork necessary to cover the client's participation in horse-related activities. The therapist needs to check each state's equine laws to see what additional information needs to be included. The horse professional should be able to help assist in gathering the appropriate release information pertaining to the horse activities.

In planning an EAP session, it is the therapist's duty to keep the horse professional informed of the issues that need to be addressed in the session. This is true for all types of therapy sessions. The therapist does not need to disclose all the details about the case to the horse professional for a successful session to occur, merely a brief summary of the goals or intentions of the next session to come. It is also good practice for the therapist and horse professional to process briefly after each session about how they felt it went and any comments or observations that were made. The treatment team meetings should help this planning process to flow more smoothly for the sessions to come.

In facilitating a session, it is the therapist's job to do the therapy and help transfer the EAP activity or experience back to life. While the horse professional is responsible for the horses and physical safety, the therapist is responsible for providing an environment that is emotionally safe and beneficial. Granted, in a balanced EAP team, the horse professional may verbalize observations and insight; nevertheless, it is the therapist's duty to facilitate the processing over the activity and application.

In addition, it is the therapist's legal and ethical duty to keep good notes on the session and to ensure that the client's rights are being respected in this process. This may take some educating by the therapist with the horse professional because many horse professionals are unfamiliar with the ethical and legal considerations of professional counseling. It is good practice for the horse professional to have notes related to the horses' behavior in the session as well and/or to sign off on the therapist's notes, all of which should be kept with the permanent file in a confidential location following the licensure laws of the state for documentation and storing of files.

Planning and Facilitating Group Sessions

All of the above information that is to be considered for individual therapy must be considered when conducting a group session as well. In addition to these guidelines, it is also important to consider the size of the group and ensure that the size is appropriate for therapeutic benefits to be maximized. Group size will be discussed in more detail in Chapter 10. Remember, thinking outside the box is not only important for the client's success but also for the success of the team. There is always more than one way to do things, so the therapist must be able to think this way as well and be creative in designing groups and activities to maximize the benefits to the clients. In group therapy, many things are often happening at once and much information is being revealed. This can be overwhelming at times to the treatment team as well as to the client; therefore, another duty of the therapist in facilitating a session is to be cautious about not focusing on too many issues or observations at once. Remember that it cannot all be resolved in one session; the main issues will continue to surface over and over until they are resolved, so don't worry about missing an opportunity. This occurs in individual therapy as well but seems to be even more apparent with groups. The treatment team may find themselves feeling overwhelmed by issues even more with groups because there are many people with issues surfacing simultaneously.

Figure 5.2
Processing can occur before, during or after an EAP activity.

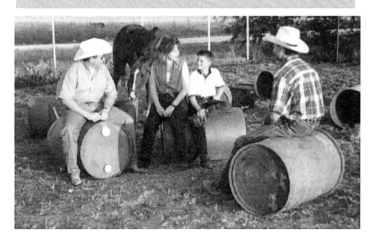

Some EAP professionals believe that the best EAP team allows the horse professional to do his/her job and the therapist sticks to the therapy. By simplifying your duties and becoming more focused, each person is able to be more effective and efficient. Others state that the longer an EAP treatment team works together, the more blurred the roles of each become – sharing in duties and roles. Nevertheless, remember that the mental health of the client is ultimately the therapist's ethical responsibility and liability. Therefore, trust within the treatment team is vital to the client's success.

Topics for Discussion:

1. *What qualifications must be met in order to operate as an EAP mental health professional?*

2. *What do you see as the most important duties of the mental health professionals in an EAP session? Discuss.*

3. *Discuss some of the ethical dilemmas that may be unique for therapists to consider when conducting EAP? Explain.*

4. *As a therapist, you are working with a horse professional who has been a school teacher. This horse person is very comfortable stepping into therapeutic questioning with the client and frequently tends to direct the course of the session. Is this a concern for you as the therapist in this team? Explain your position. Describe your approach to handling this dilemma.*

5. *You are a certified EAP horse professional interviewing for a therapist counterpart to complete your team. What characteristics would be important to you in an EAP therapist? Discuss.*

Chapter Notes

CHAPTER 5

Chapter Notes

6 THE ROLE OF THE HORSE PROFESSIONAL

Objectives:
- **Define qualifications of the EAP horse professional**
- **Explore criteria and skills of the horse professional**
- **Discuss the horse professional's role in EAP session planning**

This chapter discusses the importance of the horse professional. The horse professional's role is very pivotal in determining how much a client will be able to gain from a session. With a competent and knowledgeable horse professional, the therapist has much more freedom to be creative in working with the client on issues that arise. Minimal standards for the horse professional continue to be debated and discussed in this field; nevertheless, having expectations beyond minimum standards reap benefits without dispute.

Equine-Assisted Psychotherapy is designed as a team approach to therapy with a clinical professional and a horse professional, also referred to as an equine specialist, working together in sessions. Even if someone qualifies as both professionals, it is still highly recommended that this work be done as a team. It is safer, more effective, and more professional. These reasons will be discussed in more detail later in this chapter. Currently, as an EAP horse professional, no licensing standards exist for the equine specialists similar to the licensing standards that exist for therapists. There continues to be much discussion in the field about establishing some formal guidelines and/or standards of minimum experience and educational requirements for the equine specialist.

Many EAP professionals debate what it means to be an EAP horse professional. The question continues to be asked, "Does expertise in the equine world *via* diverse personal experience, educational classes, or certifications make you an effective EAP horse professional?" In the past, many EAP horse professionals compared themselves to a recommended point system developed by EAGALA (2006) which stated a minimum standard for EAGALA Equine Specialist. The minimum standard included experience such as work in a horse industry profession, professional/amateur competitor, degree or certification in a horse program, member of horse association, and/or horse owner. The standards were written in such a way that more than just being around horses all one's life was needed. By following these standards, the pattern emerged that the approach was attracting qualified horse people but not necessarily equipped EAP equine specialists. The standards alone prove not to be an exclusive tool for measuring EAP horse professional suitability. It is critical that a horse person wanting to do EAP must have therapeutic skills and characteristics which are often difficult to measure and/or calculate. The standards do not include specific observable qualities necessary for a safe equine specialist. So, the question remains, "What makes a good EAP horse professional?"

Experts can agree that there is more to being an effective EAP equine specialist than understanding horses. Kersten and Thomas (2004) believe that observation skills, openness, and stability are additional skills important in truly becoming a "professional." Even when guidelines from the previously described minimum standards are met, this list will not guarantee physical and/or emotional safety in every session, when using horses to assist clients with emotional issues (Kersten & Thomas, 2004). Another area that all EAP professionals agree on is that the safety of the client must be of number one importance. Therefore, high standards of professionalism, for the equine specialist as well, are in the client's best interest. If a high level of skill is not yet met, it is highly recommended that the horse professional work toward meeting professional standards before conducting EAP sessions with actual clients.

Criteria for a Safe EAP Horse Professional

As stated earlier in the chapter, meeting minimum horse experience recommendations for equine specialists does not ensure safety in an EAP session. Because EAP is professional counseling, the horse professional's duties not only include ensuring physical safety around the horses but also include being aware and conscientious of the fact that both the therapist and the horse professional play a significant role in the emotional state of the client. Remember that the entire treatment team, therapist and horse professional, are ethically responsible for doing what is in the best interest of the client.

Effective EAP horse professionals are reality-focused. They are aware of safety concerns and present them in a professional, instructive manner yet are not too rigid and inflexible. They are more in the middle of the two extremes. They understand EAP, as well as horse behavior, knowing that there is always risk involved. They don't scare clients or under-represent the capabilities of horses. They are creative, calm, aware, and demonstrate these attributes regularly (Kersten, 2004). While safety is a constant consideration, Robertson & Boyce (2008) emphasize that micro managing sessions because of safety concerns will inhibit potential learning opportunities. The perpetual challenge for the EAP equine specialist is to balance physical and emotional safety with the freedom and creativity of EAP that can lead to powerful revelation (Robertson & Boyce, 2008).

According to Hill (2012), when working with horses, there must be no confusion over who is in charge. This isn't about physical force or aggression, it's about confidence. Fortunately, no striking, biting, or kicking is necessary to settle the pecking order. With a little bit of ingenuity, the horse specialist can communicate in non-violent, effective ways with the horse. Establishing who is "in charge" starts with body language, and body language starts with one's bearing. Hill (2012) defines **bearing** as the overall manner and conduct of a person. It is a blend of attitude and physical carriage. Bearing is the air about a person, his/her outlook and manner. Just as in horse training, an effective EAP horse professional must be a confident horse handler and person. Confidence in the treatment team helps prevent physical as well as emotional injury. A confident treatment team will also generate learning and creative thinking. By being confident and reality-focused, the horse person will be more aware and productive in EAP sessions. This also translates into less stress and more enjoyable work for both the horse professional and the mental health professional (Kersten, 2004).

Tasks and Skills Needed

One of the most important duties of the horse professional is physical safety. Just as described before, being the alpha in the horse herd is paramount. In order to maximize the benefits of an EAP session, the horse professional needs to be able to move the horses and change behavior without necessarily physically touching the horse. Hill (2012) states that body language is made up of posture, position, and movement. Body language can indicate confidence, strength, and expectations or it can show uncertainty, fear, or inattentiveness. Body movements alone can suddenly stop a horse, block him from further movement, slow him down, or invite him to goof around (Hill, 2012). Since horses are basically followers. They are willing to accept guidance from the equine specialist as long as his/her intentions are clear, smooth, and confident. Horses are acutely aware of the most subtle movements, so everything the horse professional does, as the "dominant horse," sends a message to the horses whether or not that is the intention (Hill, 2012). When a horse's behavior is needing to change to ensure safety, Hill (2102) states, "use as much pressure as it takes to get the message across but as little as is needed to get the job done. The goal is subtle cueing" (p. 8). Developing a high degree of body awareness and knowing how horses read movements will help the horse professional communicate effectively with the horses in an EAP session to help provide a safer, learning environment.

As previously mentioned, there is a distinct difference between being a good "horse handler" and a good EAP "horse professional." A horse professional needs to not only be horse savvy but also good with people. Many of the characteristics of a crisis worker explained in Chapter 13 are also critical skills, techniques, and characteristics necessary for horse professionals to possess.

This combination is not easy to find. Many of the skills that make them so good with animals are the exact characteristics that make it difficult to relate to people. Nevertheless, one gifting without the other is not adequate for EAP to function at its best. Safety includes both physical as well as emotional safety in this field. The horse professional has many critical roles. In some ways, the horse professional may be the heart of a good EAP team. This person has many vital duties and responsibilities that make or break an EAP session. He/She is responsible for the safety of the clients and horses, for matching appropriate horses with clients, for helping design activities based on knowledge of horse behavior, for interpreting horse behavior to life situations, for aiding the therapist in understanding/translating horse behavior and outcomes, and for knowing the horses and being able to predict outcomes and responses. These are just a few of the key roles the horse professional plays while aiding in an EAP session.

A good EAP horse professional needs to be educated and experienced in working with and around horses. As a team member in

THE ROLE OF THE HORSE PROFESSIONAL

Equine Assisted Psychotherapy, a sound equine specialist has several qualities which enable him or her to work effectively with a licensed mental health professional. Jensen (Jensen, DeHoff, Cordero, Haveruk, & Mandrell, 2008) believes "less is more" when working with horses. It is all about communication when training. The more subtle one can be to get a conversation going, the more meaningful the conversation. The role of the equine specialist in EAP takes these same skills. Facilitating EAP is an art, and the key to success is knowing when to step in and when to step back. Haveruk (Jensen et. al., 2008) adds that this person must have a keen ability to assess potential crises quickly and calmly and can divert or intervene without removing the therapeutic value of the situation. One does this by being perceptive and sensitive to all that is happening non-verbally and by having a huge saddlebag of experiences to draw from (Jensen et. al., 2008).

Cordero (Jensen et. al., 2008) states that the EAP horse professional should be an adjunct and a compliment to the mental health professional. At the same time, the horse professional helps the client understand the role and actions of the third member of the team, the horse. The equine specialist must have a profound knowledge of horsemanship and horse characteristics and must share this information continuously with the mental health professional throughout the session for maximum therapeutic benefit. This is pivotal for the emotional and physical safety of the client and the effectiveness of the treatment process. This person must be able to decipher the body language of horses, must not be afraid of horses, and must be an observer capable of deducing what is happening with the clients without judgment (Jensen et. al., 2008).

Figure 6.1 A good EAP horse professional sees the difference between EAP and horsemanship and is willing to allow clients to tell their stories through experiences with the horses.

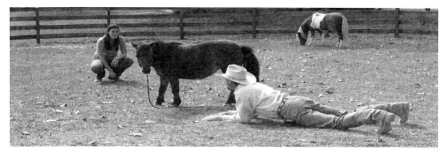

Planning an Individual Session

Planning an EAP activity for an individual session requires teamwork and communication between the therapist and the horse professional. Much of the preparation work on the horse professional's part must take place prior to the activity itself. On a regular basis, the horse person should be interacting with the horses and meeting their basic needs. This keeps the horse professional knowledgeable about the horses' responses, moods, and condition. In doing this, the equine specialist is aware of any limitations and/or concerns in horse behavior that might impact the treatment plan. It is the obligation of the EAP equine specialist to convey this information to the mental health professional as they are planning for the session. This information can be critical in the design of the activity as well as which horses will be used for the session.

The Equine Assisted Growth and Learning Association (Thomas, 2011) states that the equine specialist's role is to look for safety issues, not teach about horses. For this work to be optimally powerful, these are not "horses," they are the metaphors of what they become for the client. The client is experiencing his/her life in this session. So "ears back means they may bite" may not be relevant or meaningful to the client. The equine specialist's role as facilitator is to intervene as necessary and to do so in a way that takes into account therapeutic context, allowing for the client's interpretation and using it as a metaphoric moment while being aware of the client's physical safety (Thomas, 2011)

In order to stand back and allow the process to happen during the session, the horse professional must make sure that the facility being used for the session is free of any objects or items that could be dangerous for the horse or client during the session. The horse professional should be prepared with the appropriate props to be used in the activities. This person should have spoken with the therapist prior to the session to help design an activity based on the client's therapeutic needs.

During the session, the horse professional needs to keep his/her focus on the horse(s), observing behavior and responses while ensuring safety. Remember, it is not the horse professional's job to be a therapist. This allows the therapist to stay in therapist role to see responses and process the experience.

Planning Group Sessions

Just as with individual sessions, group sessions should be prepared for as a team. Each person has their important contributions to the success. Some unique issues for the horse professional to consider for any group/family activity are as follows: how many horses are too many, how many clients can be out with his/her horses and stay safe, safety in numbers is more challenging than safety of one person, etc.

The horse versus client ratio is a critical issue to have resolved prior to a group activity to ensure safety. After considering the therapeutic elements and criteria for determining group size, a horse professional needs to be able to speak up about how many clients should be out in an arena at one time with his/her horses. For example, let's say there are fourteen, 12-14 year old adolescents coming for a leadership workshop. What would need to be considered by the horse professional who has ten horses to choose from? Say the team agrees that therapeutically it would be most beneficial to divide the group in half and work with two groups of seven. Table 6.2 identifies three questions EAP horse professionals need to consider when setting up an equine assisted activity for a group.

Table 6.2 Questions to Consider

1. How many horses are too many to have involved?
2. Which horses will best fit the needs of the group and activity?
3. What size of space is best for this activity and number of clients/horses involved?

Horse professional need to know when there is too much activity going on to ensure safety and when they begin to recognize that they cannot see all that is going on in the arena (because there are either too many people, too many horses, or both.) These issues are critical to safety and effectiveness and should be determined prior to a session. The answer to how many clients and/or how many horses are too many may be different for different horse professionals depending on their level of confidence and experience. This decision hinges on knowledge of the horse herd and herd dynamics. Keeping in mind that no matter what arrangement is decided upon, the equine specialist must be confident in his/her position as alpha in the herd selected.

Therefore, finding what works best is key. The horse professional must know and be honest with the therapist about any personal limits in being able to maintain emotional and physical safety. A session will be much more productive with fewer horses and/or clients if that is the comfort level of the horse professional than it would be to go way beyond that limit. Facilitating beyond the horse professionals limits puts the clients in a potentially heightened unsafe situation.

In conclusion, the horse professional's role is different from that of a mental health professional for many reasons. These reasons mostly surround safety. Without quality and confident horse professionals, EAP would not be possible. The horses are the power behind this form of therapy and without professionals to help interpret our four-legged co-facilitator's input and contributions, EAP would be very limited. Therefore, it is evident that the ethical considerations that surround mental health professionals extend to the horse professionals, as well ensuring the best experience for all involved. Remember, not every horse professional is suited for EAP work; just as, not all therapists are effective with this approach.

Topics for Discussion:

1. *There has been much discussion within the field about the need for clarification as to what exactly constitutes a "horse professional" or "equine specialists." What do you think the qualifications should encompass?*

2. *What do you see as the most important duties of the horse professionals in an EAP session? Discuss.*

3. *Discuss some of the ethical dilemmas that you see that may be unique for horse professionals to consider when conducting EAP? Explain.*

4. As a horse professional, you are working with a therapist that has never been around horses before. At what point, does this factor become a concern for you? Does this ever pose any ethical concerns for the EAP team?

5. You are a certified EAP mental health professional interviewing a horse professional to team up with to conduct EAP sessions. What characteristics would be important to you in an EAP horse professional? Explain.

6. A horse kicks a client after numerous discussions from the horse professional and therapist to be aware of what messages the client is sending the horse that are irritating the horse. The client is down on the ground crying but not seriously injured. What is your response and job as a horse professional? Discuss.

CHAPTER 6

Chapter Notes

7 THE HORSE

Objectives:
- **Explore horse psychology, cues, and body language**
- **Discuss importance of horses' role in the EAP team**
- **Understand therapeutic value in horse behavior**

The history of the human race and that of the horse are closely intertwined. The human fascination with horses dates back to our caveman ancestors and, perhaps, even beyond that. Many facets of the human fascination with horses are understandable. As horses became domesticated, they became a part of survival. They were used to till fields, pull heavy loads and transport goods and passengers. Horses brought prosperity to those cultures that learned to domesticate them. Horses extended the range over which men could explore, hunt, trade, and wage war. The horse is also an important item of our social fabric. Competitions, races and games involving men and horses are as old as man's domestication of the animal itself (Miller, 1999).

Not all of our fascination with horses can be explained in practical terms. The grace and beauty of the horse enthralls us today in the same way it enthralled cavemen artists of the past. Horses are living works of art. Above all else, it is probably the mystique of the horse that so fascinates and perplexes humans. Embodied in the horse is the same range of abstract and intangible personality characteristics that we find in people. Some are fearful and others bold; some have a strong work ethic and others are lazy; some appear to have the desire to win while others are non-competitive; some react rationally to situations, others irrationally; and some always seem to be good-natured while others are hostile. Miller (1999) suggests that maybe our desire to understand the horse is nothing more than a desire to understand ourselves and the people around us.

In this chapter, we will discuss briefly the characteristics of the horse and several horse cues that play an important role in the EAP session. This information is valuable to the treatment team in order to aid them in a better understanding of their four-legged co-facilitators. With a greater understanding of the horse, the horse professional is also better able to incorporate the horse into the processing, predict behavior, and prevent potential unsafe situations.

Horse Psychology and Body Language

Like other forms of animal life, the horse is born with senses of vision, hearing, touch, smell and taste. The horse integrates its senses responding to each new stimulus with as many of them as possible (Ainslie & Ledbetter, 1980). Since horses don't communicate verbally the way people do, they rely on a highly developed combination of sensory inputs to read what is happening around them. Their senses of smell, hearing, and touch give them much information about what is happening. Horses are more capable of reading mood and intent than people may realize (Hill, 2012).

Vision

The horse's eyes are on opposite sides of the head and not in front like those of cats, humans and many dogs. Only when looking straight ahead, with its face perpendicular to the ground, can the animal direct both eyes simultaneously at the same point in space. With the horse's eyes being on the sides of its head, the horse obviously cannot see anything close to the center of its face. This is why it backs away or abruptly shifts its head, or both, when an unexpected visitor approaches the stall and delivers an overhand, downward pat to its forehead. An unerring test of a horse's trust in its handler is whether the human can place a hand directly on the animal's forehead without provoking withdrawal (Ainslie & Ledbetter, 1980).

Hearing

A horse's ears swivel on their vertical axes, somewhat like rotary antennas. When a sound provokes apprehensiveness, the horse may swing not only its head but also its entire body in the direction already taken by the ears. The ears then assume the forward, pricked position of total interest, all senses working in concert (Ainslie & Ledbetter, 1980).

Touch

Of all the marvels in its physical repertoire, none surpass the horse's sense of touch. An even slightly tense or apprehensive rider is unaware of the disturbing messages transmitted through knees, hands or seat to an increasingly impatient or demoralized horse. In contrast, the muscle language of a confident rider helps to relax and embolden a horse (Ainslie & Ledbetter, 1980). This same sensitivity is present even if interactions with the horse are on the ground.

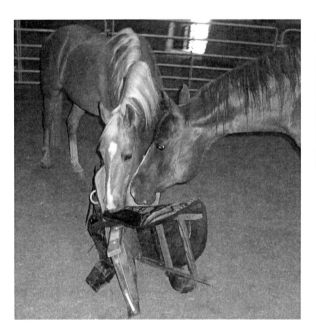

Figure 7.1
A horse will often smell and even taste new objects being investigated.

Smell

To determine whether someone or something is acceptable, the horse not only looks and listens but also does a good deal of sniffing and tasting (Ainslie & Ledbetter, 1980). For example, as depicted in Figure 7.1, the first time a horse sees a saddle; it will sniff the saddle over thoroughly and may even put the saddle leather in its mouth for further examination.

Taste

Beyond serving as a medium of identification or instrument of self-preservation (which is one in the same), the horse's sense of taste has its more festive side (Ainslie & Ledbetter, 1980). For example, horses will eat more than just grass, hay and grain. They seem to enjoy different flavors and will try just about anything once. Nevertheless, they can be selective at times as well.

Equine Needs and Attributes

Just as humans have basic needs, horses spend their time working to meet their basic needs of food, water, sleep, exercise, grooming, and space (Ainslie & Ledbetter, 1980). If they are lacking in any basic need, they are unable to perform at full capacity.

Inherent Traits

Miller (1999) summarizes ten traits found in every horse. Understanding these inbred characteristics will "unlock the secrets of horse behavior" (p. 15).

Flight. The horse in its wild state depends upon flight as its primary survival behavior. Considering its enemies and its habitat, sprinting straight away from any frightening stimulus is the best way for horses to survive. Above all else when looking to understand horse behavior, the natural instinct of this species to flee from real or imagined danger must be appreciated.

Perception. Prey species must be more perceptive than predators if they are to survive. Horses are a **prey species** that live with the danger of being eaten by their predator enemies. They are programmed to be on the lookout for danger and are always prepared to flee from it in an instant. Horses have an uncanny ability to detect sensory stimuli which are far too vague for us to sense. Miller (1999) reports that horses are incredibly aware of their surroundings, so much so that people often misinterpret the horse's reaction as "psychic" or the result of a "sixth sense" (p. 15). However, the responses, which elicit such opinions, are caused by reactions to the same five senses we possess: sight, hearing, smell, taste and touch. What is difficult for us to identify with is the superiority of those senses in the horse and the swift flight reaction that a stimulus to those senses can provoke.

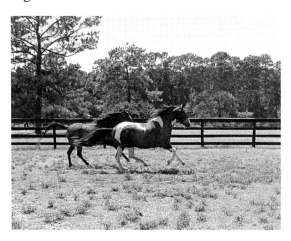

Figure 7.2
As a prey animal, a horse's innate response to uncertainty is to run away.

Response time. The horse has the fastest response time of any common domestic animal. **Response time** means the ability to perceive stimuli and react to it. This short response time is essential in a flighty creature. It isn't enough to run away. One must run away instantly and at high speed to survive.

Rapid desensitization. The horse is more quickly desensitized to frightening stimuli than any other animal. If this weren't so, horses would spend all their time running and there would be no time to meet their other basic needs. So horses, in nature, must quickly learn to ignore basically frightening but harmless things such as tumbleweeds, thunder, deer, or quail. Once they learn, they never forget.

Learning. Not only do horses desensitize faster than other domestic animals to frightening stimuli, but other kinds of learning are obtained with similar speed. If the initial experience is traumatic, the horse will henceforth fear that procedure. Conversely, if the initial experience is made pleasurable and if comfort rather than discomfort ensues, the horse will remember that and will be more accepting of such an experience in the future.

Memory. The horse's memory is nearly infallible. Horses never seem to forget anything. Fortunately, horses forgive and were it not for that fact, a majority of professional horse trainers could not make a living. The donkey and its hybrid offspring, the mule, have as keen a memory as the horse, but unlike the horse they do not forgive. Thus, donkeys and mules are notoriously more challenging to train than horses. Horses categorize every learned experience in life as something not to fear and, hence, to ignore; or something to fear and, hence, to flee. What horses experience creates lasting attitudes, especially if the horses are young (Miller, 1999).

Dr. Grandin explains that the brain of the horse stores memories as a picture, a sound, or a feeling. Occasionally, memory may be associated to a smell as well. A very common memory association is feeling. For example, a horse begins bucking when the rider changes gaits. In this instance, the saddle feels different at each gait and creates a different feeling picture in the brain (Hamilton, 2012).

Dominance hierarchy. The horse is the most easily dominated of all common domestic animals. It is a herd animal, subject to dominance hierarchy; and because it is a flight animal, the horse needs leadership to know when and where to run. In the wild, horses need leadership and readily accept it. The methods by which this can be accomplished most effectively are not natural to human beings. We must be taught (Miller, 1999). Mares are the dominant members of the wild herd. Although horses tend to associate in pairs, they demonstrate a larger loyalty to the group as a whole and, in a real sense, to the species as a whole. A newly arrived horse undergoes a period of probation, which may include physical hazing, before finding its own place in the local hierarchy. Although horses naturally prefer each other's company, they welcome human friendship at every stage of their lives from the day of birth. Moreover, when cared for by knowing persons, they flourish even if totally deprived of equine companionship (Ainslie & Ledbetter, 1980).

Movement. The horse is the only common domestic animal that exerts dominance and determines the hierarchy by controlling the movement of its peers. Dominant horses make threatening movements towards subordinate herd members. The submissive individual, yielding its space, reaffirms the role of the dominant leader. Control of movement is the basis of all horse training disciplines. Horses accept our dominance when we cause them to move when they'd prefer not to, or when we inhibit their movement (Ainslie & Ledbetter, 1980).

More specifically, a horse's feet determine where it is moving. Clinician Mark Rashid (Anderson, 2007) explains that anyone can become aware of where a horse's body is going by watching their feet. He explains that every gait, whether it's a walk, trot, canter, single-foot, or pace, has one thing in common: The barrel of the horse swings opposite the hind foot in motion as the horse takes a step. This means that when the right hind foot is stepping forward, the horse's barrel swings to the left, and when the left hind foot is stepping forward, the barrel is moving to the right.

Body language. The horse is constantly providing valuable information through body language. The horse shows what kind of mood it is in, how it is feeling physically, what it is focused on, if it understands what is being asked and much more (Hill, 2012).

Precocity. The horse is a **precocial species**, which means it is neurologically mature at birth. The imprinting period of the precocial species is immediately postpartum, when they visualize and memorize what they see move and want to follow and respect it (which in nature is usually the mother). These imprinting periods permit immediate learning and permanent retention. The best time to teach horses, therefore, is right after birth. Attitudes, temperament and reactions can be shaped in just a few hours if we know how (Miller, 1999).

Fears

Of all domestic animals, the horse is most often overcome by hysterical fright. Unfortunate experiences leave a condition imprint on the horse's brain. Ainslie and Ledbetter (1980) describe seven different situations horses may experience that in general result in a fear response.

Loss of Balance. Because it is helpless against attack when off its feet, a healthy horse only lies down if it feels safe. For the same reason, it hesitates to risk loss of balance on unfamiliar footing.

The Unfamiliar. Until satisfied that something new is harmless, a horse tends to assume that it may be dangerous. The horse displays comparable apprehensiveness in a new environment or when startled by an unfamiliar sound, smell, or appearance of an unfamiliar moving object.

Predators. A domesticated horse may never have seen a snake or a big cat in its life but is sure to fear either on first sight.

The Poll Bone. This is a loose bone between the ears. If struck with force, it can penetrate the brain and kill the horse. Instinctively protective of this vulnerable spot, horses may become frantic when led toward a low-roofed van or trailer, particularly if they have hit their heads on one before.

Water. Horses rarely learn to love swimming and seldom enter deep water for the first time without great apprehensiveness.

Death. Horses are reluctant to approach a decomposing carcass, the scent of which is more apparent to them than to their riders. They probably associate all death with predatory attack, fearing that the killer may still be near.

Remembered Fears. If a horse has not been helped to overcome a fear, it will forever after be rattled, or worse, when confronted by the cause of the fear. The more often the experience is repeated and corrective measures are omitted, the deeper and more difficult the problem becomes.

Curiosity

The horse's curiosity is as keen as that of the cat or raccoon, and its need to satisfy the feeling is no less acute. For instance, one way to get an unfamiliar horse to approach is for you to turn your back to the horse, be very still and pretend to be indifferent. Few horses can resist such a curiosity (Ainslie & Ledbetter, 1980).

Playfulness

The spirit of fun persists with age and growth. It is a key factor in the successful schooling of a horse. The young horse that is allowed to regard work as fun learns its skills most rapidly and applies them most willingly. When opportunities for play are sparse, the animal devises games of its own. It plays with objects in its stall, and it often invents pastimes with which to bother human beings. A horse's favorite playmate is another horse (Ainslie & Ledbetter, 1980).

Boredom and Frustration

The nature of the horse is that of a browser. It does best with daily changes of scene. It wants to poke its nose into things, to feel different textures beneath its feet and see different sights. If deprived of new stimuli, a horse becomes bored and frustrated, even when given ample exercise under saddle (Ainslie & Ledbetter, 1980).

Comprehension

Horses understand each other very well. Equine comprehension of human wishes is even more impressive. Unless the horse is an unusually dull animal or has been turned off by mistreatment, it understands the words that describe the gaits and other physical maneuvers of its work. It understands other words that refer to aspects of its behavior. It understands and reacts to tones of voice. Another element of equine comprehension resembles our own sense of injustice. A human being arouses jealousies among paddocked horses by offering more friendly attention to one over the others. If the other horse has enjoyed the person's attention in the past and has come to expect it, it may become jealous. It may crowd the new favorite and, if still frustrated, may try to nip the human visitor.

Horse Cues

From ears, eyes and mouth to legs, feet and tail is a vast expanse. If we linger too long at the ears, we may miss the whole recital. Similarly, if we yield to human instinct and dwell too deeply on the horse's vocal utterances, we are lost. The snorts, knickers, neighs, whinnies, bellows, squeals and screams of horses are meaningful only in conjunction with the body language of the moment or the situation of the moment, or both. The sounds are best understood as punctuation marks or emphases (Ainslie & Ledbetter, 1980).

In general, there are several nonverbal cues that all equine exhibit when in different situations or feeling different emotions. An awareness of these cue themes or trends is valuable to the EAP team's approach to a session and to diffuse safety incidents before they arise.

CHAPTER 7

Ainslie and Ledbetter (1980) include a list of common horse emotions and expressions that are beneficial for the EAP team to consider.

The Happy Horse

In a moment of particular enjoyment, the horse drops its head and then flips it high and completes a full, skyward circle with its nose. Its behavior is eager, interested, alert, playful and responsive. A raised tail is the primary sign of playfulness.

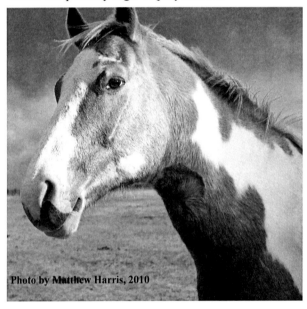

Figure 7.3 Based on observation of eyes and ears, head and neck posture, what cues is this horse giving you which can help you predict future behavior?

The Proud Horse

When thoroughly pleased with itself and the prevailing situation, the horse registers it satisfaction by prancing with ears straight forward, nostrils flaring, tail up, head pointed downward on arched neck.

The Interested Horse

The interested horse stands with its nose, eyes and ears pointed straight ahead at the object of interest, and the animal moves its body directly into line, if allowed.

The Eager Horse

The eager horse shows impatience by stamping a front foot. And then a hind foot. It shakes his head. It dances sideways. The horse's behavior is often confused with that of nervousness. But he is not actually unruly and is nervous only in the keyed-up way of good performers before they take the stage.

The Healthy Horse

A healthy horse's glowing coat reflects a lot of light. Mane and tail are soft rather than matted, lumpy or coarse. It tends to be playful, responsive to attention and interested in everything. Its hooves are strong.

The Bored Horse

A bored horse shifts its weight restlessly from foot to foot. It holds its head sleepily downward for a while and then moves it actively, with much ear motion-hunting up something of interest. Or it may nip a horse to arouse it or perhaps to alarm the human beings and get something started. Bored horses are extremely mouthy.

The Submissive Horse

A horse might demonstrate submissiveness by assuming a suckling posture, working their mouths like nursing foals. This seldom is seen in older horses except in extreme stress (Ainslie & Ledbetter, 1980).

The Bereaved Horse

A bereaved horse spends some of its time moving around its stall in restless circles, and much more with its head out the door, ears pricked forward, looking in whatever direction the longed-for companion was last seen. The horse constantly sniffs the air for the missing scent. It frequently utters long, nickering calls. If the separation is more than brief, the horse goes off its feed, loses sleep and does its work poorly. In the same plight, a pastured horse spends its time racing up and down beside the fences, looking and calling.

The Frightened Horse

Apprehensiveness. When apprehensive, the horse directs full attention at the object of concern. Ears, nose and eyes point straight at it, although the head may swing slightly, or the animal may step sideways for sensory focus at different angles. A good deal of loud sniffing is probable. Furrows appear over the eyes, giving them an appearance of anxiety that is completely recognizable when combined with the rest of the body language. Occasionally, the horse withdraws its head, with neck highly arched. The horse becomes light-footed, dancing restlessly in place.

Thorough Fright. A horse does not willingly tolerate prolonged fear. To rid itself of the sense of menace, it tries to flee. Its instinctive wish is to rear on the hind legs, pivot and rush away. Its tail becomes still. The horse plants its feet and at the slightest opportunity spins away. The horse is now completely awash in sweat. The whites of its rolling, frightened eyes are probably visible.

Total Panic. When in total panic, a horse's eyes glaze. It screams. If it now breaks loose, it may try to go through a barn wall. Or it may tear itself to pieces on a barbed-wire fence. Or it may collapse in shock, falling flat on the ground, where it lays shaking from head to toe and breathing heavily. Panic expended, the horse is in a state of nervous exhaustion. It stands with feet widely sprawled in an effort to maintain vertical balance, head almost to the ground, eyes closed, ears flopped down motionless to the sides, body quivering, scarcely breathing.

The Angry Horse

Irritation. The ears lie back lightly. The tail swishes to one side, as if at a fly. The hindquarters tense, ready to kick.

Greater Irritation. The ears lie closer to the skull. The tail motion is more vigorous on one side. The rear hoof on that side now raises slightly off the ground.

Thorough Irritation. The ears are now pinned down. The tail lashes from side to side. The eyes flash anger. The horse kicks straight back at the source of irritation.

Outright Anger. The tail whistles horizontally, moving quickly enough to cut human skin and draw blood. Occasionally, the tail pops straight up and down, slapping against the rear. The head turns toward the object of anger, ears pinned, upper lip curled or quivering (a sign of intent to bite), eyes a glare and taking dead aim. Having zeroed in, the horse shifts its weight to the front and kicks with both hind legs.

In summary, anxious movement as seen in a frightened and possibly angry horse are often heralded by a subtle shift in expression, body language, or breathing. As listed in Figure 7.4, Hill (2012) identifies the following behaviors that indicate a horse is uncomfortable, afraid, or confused (p. 10).

Figure 7.4. Signs of Anxiety

- Trying to escape – moving feet away from person or thing
- Leaning away or swerving away
- Reaching toward with head, ears pinned, and nose forward
- Turning hindquarters toward someone
- Raising or lowering head swiftly
- Flattening ears
- Shaking head
- Switching tail
- Clamping tail
- Rearing
- Bucking
- Kicking
- Striking
- Bolting
- Raising a leg
- Pulling away
- Holding breath
- Wide eyed
- Snorting sharply
- Screaming
- Pawing
- Backing away

Application to EAP

With regard to Equine-Assisted Psychotherapy, a thorough understanding and appreciation for horse behavior and cues aids in the therapy process on multiple levels. First of all, it is important to acknowledge the role of the third member of the treatment team. Without the horse, EAP would resemble play therapy in a giant sandbox. The horses' job in this work is to be themselves. In order to utilize the third member in the treatment team most effectively, it is vital for the equine specialist to be aware of the subtle cues of the horse. More specifically, it is critical to be sensitive to the cues that relate to flight instinct, fear, and anger response. With this awareness, the equine specialist is better able to gauge when a release of pressure is necessary to regulate potential safety concerns. With a keen eye for the cues that lead up to the kick, bite, and/or lunge, an equine specialist can allow situations to flow without a dramatic intervention. Randy Mandrell, advanced equine-specialist, states, "The key to safety in a session is not just knowing when your horse is about to kick or bite, but rather knowing what your horse does two-to-three warnings prior to the kick or bite. Those are the warning signs you need to pay attention to. With that, you can begin to adjust and discuss with the therapist about how to release pressure if the clients don't back off on their own. I usually will check in with the clients at that point to see if they were aware of what was going on for the horse (Mandrell, personal communication, Jan. 2011)." Hill (2012) refers to this as **pre-cues**. A pre-cue is given just a second before the cue to allow the horse to gather himself mentally and physically. Think of the pre-cue as the sign of what is to come.

In addition, the physical, mental, and social needs of a horse are very similar to the needs of humans. Understanding the horse in this sense gives the EAP team valuable information for therapy. Many metaphors can be drawn from the similarities between horse and human behavior, as well as treatment goals reached through the process of helping a horse who has been deprived of a basic need, just as therapists might with their client. This gives clients an opportunity to be an active participant in the treatment plan and outcomes for the horse, which in turn results in growth and learning for clients.

Horse behavior provides a non-verbal description of their thoughts and intentions. It is important for the equine specialist to be a translator of this non-verbal language for safety reasons. However, it is not important that this language be taught to the client. The power of the horses in this team is that their actions can be interpreted by the clients in very diverse ways. The interpretations can vary as much as our clients themselves vary. What is important is that through the raw interaction with these horses, the clients are learning about themselves, their belief systems, their choices, and relationships. The horses provide a mirror at times to help the clients look at their behavior in a new way. This concept will be discussed in more details in the chapters to come. As a result, knowledge of the horse psychology is a prerequisite for the equine specialist facilitating this work; however, the clients' understanding of the psychology is not necessary.

Topics for Discussion:

1. Discuss how a horse professional's knowledge of horse behavior can positively impact the process in an EAP session? When might this knowledge be detrimental to therapy?

2. Discuss how horse professionals' knowledge of horse behavior can reduce safety concerns- both physical and emotional safety.

3. When you see one of your horse's anger level increasing, what is your response? At what point do you intervene in the EAP session? Discuss what this intervention might look like.

4. What are the pros and cons to having a therapist who is also very knowledgeable about horse behavior?

Chapter Notes

8 WHO CAN BENEFIT

Objectives:
- **Determine when EAP is therapeutically beneficial**
- **Define EAP versus EAL**
- **Compare various client structures**
- **Explore client issues and diagnoses often addressed in EAP**

Today more than ever, mental-health practitioners are being challenged to develop new strategies for both preventing and treating psychological problems (Corey, 1995). In this chapter, we will discuss these various therapy structures in more detail revealing the benefits and functions of each format. Equine-Assisted Psychotherapy is appropriate in various formats such as for individuals, groups, and/or families desiring help with behavioral, relational, spiritual, emotional, and/or habitual issues.

Equine-assisted growth and learning serves a number of functions. It includes both Equine-Assisted Psychotherapy (EAP) as well as Equine-Assisted Learning (EAL). It can be used as an enrichment experience in leadership development or as a teambuilding activity for participants who define themselves as "well functioning." In these cases, Equine-Assisted Learning (EAL) has the potential to enhance relationships, accentuate strengths, and normalize concerns about negotiating life transitions (Clapp & Rudolph, 1993). In addition, EAP can be used as a component of therapy to enhance therapeutic results and/or serve as a tool for assessing and gathering additional information about the participants' patterns of interaction. Finally, EAP can also be used exclusively as a short-term therapeutic intervention for those experiencing various levels of distress. The information clients learn about themselves can help them define and clarify problem areas and treatment goals, can help them find solutions to current life issues, and can motivate them to use therapy again in the future (Clapp & Rudolph, 1993).

The definitions of EAP and EAL are distinctly similar (see Table 8.1). These terms are labels intended to describe a type of service being provided. Whether you focus on providing psychotherapy, learning, coaching, counseling, or educational services, the label which best fits for the type of service being provided is chosen. Nevertheless, this book will focus on the term "EAP" throughout. The model and standards remain the same, no matter the service. The differentiation lies in the population to be served, the goals and objectives of the session, and the focus of facilitation agreed upon by goals (EAGALA, 2012).

Table 8.1 Definition of EAP and EAL

Equine Assisted Psychotherapy (EAP) incorporates horses experientially for emotional growth and learning. It is a collaborative effort between a mental health professional and a horse professional working with the client and horses to address treatment goals.

Equine Assisted Learning (EAL) incorporates horses experientially for growth and learning. It is a collaborative effort between a mental health professional, horse professional, and other specialized professionals working with the clients and horses to address learning goals.

EAGALA (2012)

Client Structures

Individual Therapy

Individual counseling is one type of client structure frequently used. Using EAP with individuals is very impactful for many clients. One example is the challenging client that "knows the counseling lingo" and has been in the system so long that he/she knows the "right" answers but are not able to live by them. In this situation, EAP forces the client out of his/her comfort zone and into new territory where words don't hold much power. Actions hold the power. This requires the individual to make changes rather than just talk about them. This format allows the client to observe where those changes need to be made in life and to experience the results. The age of the client and the nature of the activity will determine how much verbal processing is necessary for the client to be able to generalize the experience to life.

To lessen larger safety concerns and the fear element in using horses, the EAP team should start out very basic in the client's initial work with a horse. In other words, do not just rush into getting them on the horse. In fact, as a general rule that is discouraged. EAP is not horsemanship. Many experts in the field believe that groundwork allows for maximum therapeutic benefits to occur. For instance, the Equine-Assisted Growth and Learning Association (EAGALA) has gone so far as to base their EAP model exclusively on groundwork experiences (EAGALA, 2012). Many of the first sessions should be introductory and assessment focused -- introducing the client to the horse and the horse to the client. There is no set formula or order of activities in this work. Progression in each session is determined by the client's needs and goals. Nevertheless, one approach to an individual introductory session could be using the "select a horse" technique explained in Table 8.2. This is effective with a variety of clients and can have increasing intensity when using horses that are more difficult to catch and/or working in larger areas.

Family Therapy

Every aspect of Equine-Assisted Psychotherapy is exciting, challenging and enlightening. Family therapy is no exception. After the EAP team has had several successful family sessions, a therapist seldom goes back to conventional office therapy.

Bradshaw (1996) discusses the importance of fulfilling family needs. According to Bradshaw, family needs include a sense of worth, a sense of physical security or productivity, a sense of intimacy and relatedness, a sense of unified structure, a sense of responsibility, a need for challenge, stimulation, a sense of joy, affirmation and spiritual grounding. In family EAP sessions, the lack of fulfillment in one or all of these needs is often present. A properly planned family EAP session naturally addresses and challenges these needs.

Many of the family activities are similar to individual and group techniques as seen in Table 8.3. Lack of creative thinking is the only limit to adding and developing one's own session techniques (Kersten & Thomas, 1999).

Table 8.2 Sample Individual Activity

Description: Select a Horse

Type: Individual, family, or group

Objective: Assessment to evaluate client's behavior and responses

Set up:
1. This can be done in an arena, round pen, or pasture. The number of horses does not matter, although it can be useful to have multiple horses to add to the dynamics of the horse herd and provide the client(s) opportunities for choice. Various tools could be lying around (i.e. halters, props) or not!
2. Ask the client to choose a horse(s) and bring him (them) back here or to another spot as defined by facilitators or the client (i.e. "Select a horse or horses and take them to where they feel most comfortable.")

Observations and Possible Discussion Questions:
1. How does the client react to the instructions?
2. How does the client approach the horses, and how do the horses respond? What are the client's reactions to the horses' responses (quit, get frustrated, try new ideas, ask for help, etc.)?
3. What are the moments where shifts/changes occur in the client's and horses' behaviors? How do these changes in turn affect the responses of client/horses? What worked, what didn't work?
4. Where is the client's focus at various times? What is their non-verbal language communicating?
5. Which horse does the client choose and why? Does s/he stick with that horse or change, and why? What are the other horses doing while the client is focused on a specific horse? What are the horses' dynamics with each other?
6. How does this relate to human interactions (such as meeting someone for the first time)?
7. With the various feelings, thoughts, and reactions that occurred, who or what does the horse(s) remind the client of in his/her life?

EAGALA (2006)

Table 8.3 – Sample Family Therapy Activity

Description: Temptation Alley or Metaphor Alley

Objective: Teamwork, communication, problem solving, dealing with addictions (or a family member with addictions) or other temptations and stressors, overcoming challenges, roles and responsibilities. This can function as an assessment of family dynamics and provide an intervention to make needed changes in those dynamics.

Set up:
1. Build an alleyway and fill it with various obstacles (inside the alleyway and on the outside edges of the alleyway) and temptations (hay, grain, carrots, etc.). Note: You can also ask the clients to build the alleyway and enhance the metaphors by having the family name each of the items as obstacles/temptations in their lives.
2. You will need one horse, a halter and two or more lead ropes of various sizes, types, and strengths (i.e. long line, short line, yarn, etc.)

Two person activity:
1. Ask the clients to each attach a rope to the halter.
2. Explain to the couple that their goal is to lead this horse through the alleyway with the following rules:
a. The horse can not leave the alleyway
b. The horse can not knock anything over
c. The horse can not eat anything
d. The couple can not go into the alleyway
e. The couple can not move or knock anything over
f. The couple will each have a lead rope - they can hold on to the far end of the lead rope with one hand only (they can switch hands quickly if needed, but no double grabbing)
3. Ask the couple to decide on a consequence if any of the 6 violations above occur - the consequence is something to be done right here and now - so that when a violation occurs, they stop and do the consequence, then move on.
4. Optional - invite the couple to walk through the alleyway first before starting.

OR: Ask the clients to get the horse(s) through their metaphor (what the alley represents) without placing any rules, etc.

Three or more people variation:
Same as two person, but each person picks a rope and attaches it to the horse, or do not use any ropes at all.

Observations and Possible Discussion Questions:
1. If the clients built their own alleyway – what were the horses' behaviors and responses to what they built during that process? Invite the clients to share what they built.
2. What are the roles and dynamics of the individuals and horse? How does the couple/family communicate? Where do they physically place themselves in relation to each other and the horse (i.e. one leading in front, and the other behind, are they able to see each other, etc.)? Where do each focus?
3. How does the horse respond/feel throughout the activity? Who or what might the horse be for them?

> 4. What are the difficult moments and why? Where in the alleyway do those occur?
> 5. What are the smoothest moments and why? Where in the alleyway do those occur?
> 6. How does the consequence affect the individuals, horse, and process?
> 7. What worked/didn't work and does that happen at home?
>
> Variations: Be creative with your alleyway! If facilitators build the alleyway, add additional metaphor ideas, such as an area of the alleyway that is too wide for the ropes to reach (gives the metaphor of being at the end of your rope): how do they get through? The possibilities and metaphors are endless! Have various types of props around the clients may choose to use.
>
> EAGALA (2006)

Group Therapy

Professional counselors create various groups to fit special needs. In fact, the types of groups that can be designed are limited only by one's creativity. Groups can be used for either therapeutic or educational purposes or for a combination of the two. Some groups deal primarily with helping people make fundamental changes in their ways of thinking, feeling, and behaving. Other groups, with an educational focus, teach members specific coping skills (Corey, 1995). Using EAP with groups seems to magnify the group dynamics and interactions forcing the participants to grow in social skills, communication skills, teamwork, leadership and cooperation.

Group activities are closely related to family techniques and activities. The difference, of course, is that groups are connected by situations more than being connected by family ties. The definition of **group therapy** is "a form of treatment where a group of clients are treated together." The therapist uses the emotional interactions of the group members to help them get relief from distress and modify their behavior (Leong & Tinsley, 2008). The group members themselves participate in their own treatment as well as assisting in other members' treatment. Group therapy techniques are useful and effective with many groups such as children, adolescents, and/or parents. A sample group EAP activity is described in Table 8.4.

Remember, there are limitless ways that groups, families, and individuals can successfully complete these activities. Yet, to be successful requires employing certain healthy skills such as nonverbal and verbal communication, assertiveness, creative thinking, problem-solving, leadership, taking responsibility, work, confidence, positive attitude, teamwork and relationships. It is always interesting and fun to watch and see how participants finally succeed (Kersten and Thomas, 1999).

Table 8.4a – Sample Group Activity

Description: Life's Obstacles/Jumps/Goals (whatever metaphor fits)

Type: Individual, Family, Group

Objective:
    This activity is probably the most widely used for groups. It can be used as an assessment for an initial session or as an intervention tool in later sessions. It addresses issues such as teamwork, communication, problem-solving, relationships, leadership, overcoming challenges, boundaries, attitude, and definitions/expectations.

Set up:
1. Prior to starting (before the clients arrive), place various props inconspicuously around the edges of the arena - i.e. poles and cones.
2. One or multiple horses may be used, although multiple horses are preferable because of the additional dynamics they add.
3. Set up a jump in the middle of the arena.
4. Explain to the clients that their goal is to get a horse to go over the jump. (Note: the jump can be labeled as an obstacle the group is trying to overcome).

Variation: Incorporate additional rules. Be sure that any rule added is therapeutically meaningful. The treatment team must discuss about areas of extreme responses that exploration in that area may uncover further awareness or understanding of situation. (i.e. notice group is using physical touch as only means to communicate to horses and would like to explore group's ability to communicate when physical touch is not allowed)

5. Let the group know that, as in life, there are certain rules they must follow:
    a. NO physically touching the horse(s) in any way whatsoever - including throwing things or using things that touch them.
    b. NO bribing or simulating bribing (pretending to have treats).
    c. NO verbally talking (they may use horse noises to the horses). (Optional: You may give them a very limited time to plan).
6. Optional: Ask the group to decide on a consequence if any of those rules are broken (consequence is to be done here and how – stop what they are doing, do the consequence and move on).

CHAPTER 8

Table 8.4b – Sample Group Activity, cont.

Observations and Possible Discussion Questions:

1. How does the group communicate at various points – to each other and with the horses? What are the responses of horses/humans?
2. What roles do each person and horse play?
3. What are some patterns of the group/horses?
4. How are decisions made, and what are the reactions of the group members?
5. When things get challenging, frustrating, or emotional, how does each respond?
6. When do changes/shifts occur in the behaviors of people and horses? What brings about those changes? What ideas/resources do they employ?
7. What are the reactions of the group members to each other and the horses? What are the horses' reactions to them and what is the group doing in those moments?
8. Where are the group members and horses physically located and focused in moments that seem difficult or that seem to work?
9. How do the rules/consequences play a part in the process? How are they defined, and where do the group members focus – on limitations or opportunities?
10. How does each member of the group respond to the "success?" How is "success" defined for each person (watch non-verbal and verbal responses)?

EAGALA (2006)

Issues Often Addressed in EAP

Participants learn how to communicate non-verbally with the horses and see how their behavior greatly affects their relationship with the horses. The participants are involved in many activities with the horses which require participants to work together, communicate, problem-solve, and be creative. By doing this, the participants quickly see what works and what does not work. Participants discuss how the activities, relationships, and interactions with the horses are metaphors for life experiences and dealing with family, friends, and other people. Through all activities, the key issues that are most frequently targeted and discussed deal with:

- self-confidence & attitude
- teamwork
- boundaries & trust

- fears & safety
- communication
- peer pressure
- personalities and respect
- conflict resolution
- anger management
- creativity in problem solving
- breaking bad habits

The EAP approach may not be an ideal fit for all clients, therapists or health professionals. Nevertheless, the success deeply depends upon the treatment team's ability to rely on the horse as a legitimate, dependable member of the treatment team as well as the team's creativity. To list a few, EAP has been found to be highly effective with the following behavioral and mental health issues:

- Abuse & Neglect
- Anger management
- Attention Deficit (ADD/ADHD)
- Autism spectrum
- Behavior problems
- Depression & Anxiety
- Eating Disorders
- Grief
- Parenting
- Post Traumatic Stress Disorder
- Reactive Attachment Disorder
- Substance Abuse & Chemical Dependency
- Marriage, Family, and other Relational issues

Common Fears and Misconceptions of Clients

Spending time with horses, whether it be riding, leisure, and/or sport, can be beneficial mentally, emotionally, physically, and spiritually. Nevertheless, EAP is not about recreation or riding. Many clients come in with the false expectation that EAP will involve horsemanship. It is important to inform the client(s) on what to expect in this therapeutic process. Specifically, EAP focuses on human skills, not horse skills. Horsemanship is about the instructor directing specific skills with horses. EAP is about the clients being themselves. In addition, treatment goals, objectives, and interventions are identified and documented. Sessions are structured and facilitated to deliberately address the reasons clients are coming to therapy. The activities in sessions are designed to best create metaphors to "real life." This allows for metaphorical learning as everything done with the horses is related to what is happening at home, school, work, and in relationships (EAGALA, 2012). Many times in this process, clients may struggle with finding their own solutions and want someone to tell them every step. For example, it may take time for the clients to become comfortable with the idea of finding their own solution to putting the halter on rather than being told the "proper" way to halter a horse. The therapeutic value in allowing that process to happen possibly could be metaphorical for discovery of how to halter the "fear" in their life or how to halter "whatever issue" brought them to therapy. One solution may look different than another solution. Does that make either solution wrong or just different?

Clients new to EAP and unfamiliar with horses tend to be most often afraid of the horse itself. One client I worked with was so terrified of the horse that it took about three sessions before she would even touch the horse. Many clients have the misconception that when a horse makes eye contact, the horse is threatening them and may become aggressive toward them, even if unprovoked. Because clients are more familiar with dog behavior, they often treat the horse as if it were a dog. With this response comes many fears associated with predator behavior.

An even greater and more universal fear for participants in EAP experience is that of looking foolish. Many times, participants will not try some options or ideas because they fear they will look foolish in front of others. Again, this apprehension is one to be explored and often used in the therapy process. Most often, this fear is representative of a similar fear in their life, based on a false belief that leads to a fear of rejection. If this fear manifests frequently in the arena, this pattern is most often present in life as well.

The misconceptions and fears regarding this work can all be information about the client. Do not disregard their response, ask about it. Ask about how these fears and misconceptions look in their life? Do they find themselves fearful or disillusioned by other situations and/or people in their live? Most importantly, these reactions and beliefs can be therapeutic issue arising so be mindful of your response to this.

Figure 8.5 The horse's response to a client varies from client to client. The horse responds in-the-moment based on information presented by the client.

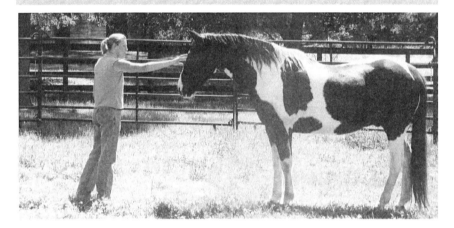

Case Summary

One of the sessions that always stands out most in my mind when discussing fears and misconceptions is a round-penning and halter activity with one of our therapy horses named "Cody." Cody was abused by a past owner and struggles with trust and fears related to people. He always helps clients face their fears and see them from a different perspective. Cody, himself, creates some fears within the clients because they are not sure how he will respond. Just his story alone, scares them. Cody is always a challenge to touch and very difficult to halter. Nevertheless, it can be done. The interesting part of working with Cody is in how close he will let them get. The client who has not yet resolved his/her own fears is unable to get close because Cody runs away. With clients who are still hiding their issues and not honest about the struggles they are facing, Cody charges toward and challenges. Neither client is able to halter Cody. Nevertheless, as the clients work through many of the issues and develops more confidence and assertiveness, they are able to touch him. I am always amazed at the parallels with regard to timing as to when the client is able to actually halter him. Without fail, this happens at the time when the clients feel they have worked through and resolved the issues at hand. What a great finale this is – the clients are able to physically halter this horse that has multiple fears and at the same time the clients feel like they have finally gotten a grip on personal fears. This is always a very empowering and reassuring moment for clients.

In conclusion, Equine-Assisted Psychotherapy is an experiential modality of mental health treatment, growth, and learning. It involves setting up activities (representing life opportunities) with horses which will require the client, family, or group to apply certain skills and awareness. Non-verbal communication, assertiveness, creative thinking and problem-solving, leadership, work, taking responsibility, teamwork and relationships, confidence, and attitude are several examples of the tools utilized and developed through this approach (EAGALA, 2012). Overall, EAP is a highly effective therapeutic approach that has proven life-changing for many.

Topics of Discussion:

1. *Discuss the pros and cons to individual, family, and group EAP.*

2. *Define EAP and EAL. What is the difference between the two?*

3. *Pick three behavioral and/or mental issues that EAP can benefit and discuss reasons why this form of therapy is beneficial.*

4. *Create an activity that could be used with a group. Include a name, description, objective and setup, along with discussion questions.*

5. Discuss safety concerns that would be unique to working with a group in EAP versus working with an individual in an EAP session.

Chapter Notes

Chapter Notes

9 WORKING WITH SPECIFIC AGE GROUPS

Objectives:
- **Evaluate who will most benefit from this form of therapy**
- **Explain stages of development and their role in designing EAP sessions**
- **Identify how age plays a role in EAP**
- **Discuss the importance of the treatment team's knowledge and awareness of cognitive and psychosocial development**

Although Equine-Assisted Psychotherapy is a highly effective therapeutic choice, it is not suited for all clients and/or all therapists. Within the field, it has been argued that EAP requires a certain degree of cognitive development before the full benefit can be reached. The client's developmental maturity influences the means to which the client can process the information from the session. Knowing this, the treatment team is responsible for tailoring EAP activities to be age and developmentally appropriate.

In this chapter, we will review Piaget's stages of cognitive development and Erikson's stages of psychosocial development. This overview will explore the important components of human development from birth to adulthood and explain the changes in cognitive processing as a person transitions through these stages. Generally, people pass through the stages at similar ages unless the process has been interrupted or slowed down due to issues such as trauma, illness, learning disabilities, or genetics. We will explore the reasons why the EAP team needs to be aware of these developmental stages in relation to their client.

Piaget's Cognitive Developmental Theory

Cognitive development refers to the development of various mental activities such as perceiving, remembering, reasoning, and problem solving. Jean Piaget (1970, 1972) provided the most insight into cognitive development as a result of his years of research. By mistake, Piaget discovered an interesting phenomenon about child development. The mistakes made by many children of the same age were often strikingly similar (and strikingly different from those made by children of other stages). It occurred to Piaget that children's cognitive strategies are age-related, and that the way children think about things changes with age regardless of the specific nature of what they are thinking about (Crooks & Stein, 1991). Piaget believed that we learn to understand our world as we constantly adapt and modify our mental structures through assimilation and accommodation. As we develop, assimilation allows us to maintain important connections with the past while accommodation helps us to adapt and change as we gain new experiences (Crooks & Stein, 1991).

Pastorino & Doyle-Portello (2010) explain Piaget's cognitive-developmental stages: sensorimotor, preoperational, concrete operational and formal operational and describes the achievements of each stage.

Sensorimotor Stage (birth to 24 months)

The sensorimotor stage consists of six sub-periods during infancy which comprise practical intelligence – action knowledge. Neonates and young infants do not understand objects unless they are experiencing the object through the senses: touching, holding, seeing, hearing, tasting or smelling. During this stage, the child does not understand that milk is milk; they simply understand the taste, temperature, and smell that they eventually connect with satisfying hunger as they develop.

Preoperational Stage (approximately 2 to 6 or 7 years)

The preoperational stage marks the beginning of thought and the marvelous prelogical intellectual antics associated with early childhood. The preoperational child centers on only one element of a situation at a time, though many details may be noticed in rapid succession. This child is now able to perform mental actions such as imagination, memory, and symbolization. At this stage, the child recognizes a bottle of milk and associates it with satisfying hunger and comfort. The most powerful of the functions in this stage is development of language, which provides the user with both a ready-made system of symbols for relating to objects and for socializing though through communicative interactions with others. For example, the child understands the word milk and utters the same sounds when pointing at the object. This illustrates a final point about this stage -- the introduction of thought processing known as abstract thinking. While levels of abstract thinking progress in concert with the stages, the ability to think abstractly is the very hallmark of symbolic thought achieved at the preoperational stage.

Concrete Operational Stage (6 or 7 to 12 years, but may last through adulthood)

The concrete operational stage signals the beginning of cognitive operations in relation to concrete objects. The term concrete refers to the child's ability to cognize and operates on elements of physical reality that can be experienced. It is not required that these elements be physically present and manipulable; what is important is that the elements be capable of being physically experienced or imagined.

Formal Operational Stage (approximately 12 years through adulthood)

In the formal operational stage, the individual becomes capable of operating mentally on hypotheses and propositions, some of which may be contrary to fact. Whereas the concrete operational thinker reasons in terms of concrete experiences, the formal operational thinker reasons in terms of possibilities. These possibilities are not arbitrary imaginings or fantasies freed of cognitive constraints or objectivity. Rather, such possibilities entail the logical permutation of potential realities and the consideration of "if…then" logical relationships.

Erikson's Psychosocial Stages of Development

In addition to Piaget's developmental stages, Erikson's psychosocial stages are also useful to the EAP team. Psychoanalyst Erik Erikson emphasized the importance of psychosocial development throughout the life-span. Erikson's major contribution to psychology centers around the idea that people continue to change and differentiate through middle age and into their senior years as they encounter various rites of passage (Erikson, 1950; Davison & Neale, 1998; & Feldman, 2008). Erikson follows human development from infancy through late adulthood, noting the psychosocial crisis and major developments of each stage.

Berger (2012) describes the eight stages of Erikson's psychosocial development to include the following:

Infancy (approximate age 0-1)

The infant must learn the difference between ***trust and mistrust***. In the caregiver-baby relationship, the infant develops a sense of trust or mistrust that basic needs such as nourishment, warmth, cleanliness, and physical contact will be provided.

Early Childhood (approximate age 2-3)

The toddler must work to master his/her physical environment to learn the difference between ***autonomy and doubt.*** During this stage, children learn self-control as a means of being self-sufficient (i.e. toilet training, feeding, walking, or developing shame and doubt about their abilities to be autonomous).

Play age (approximate age 3-6)

The play age child works on developing conscience, sexual identity; and how to initiate actions, not simply imitate others. The preschooler's objective is to learn the difference between ***initiative and guilt***. During this stage, children are anxious to investigate adult activities, but may also have feelings of guilt about trying to be independent and daring.

School-aged child (approximate age 7-11)

The school-aged child develops knowledge of the difference between ***industry and inferiority***, further developing a sense of self-worth by refining skills. During this stage, children learn about industry -- imagination, curiosity, and other learning skills. Otherwise, they develop feelings of inferiority if they fail, or if they think they fail, to master tasks.

Adolescence (approximate age 12-18)

The adolescent struggles with ***identity versus identity confusion*** (role confusion). During this stage, adolescents try to figure out who they are, how they are unique, if they want to have a meaningful role in society, how they can establish sexual, ethnic, and career identity. Feelings of confusion can arise over these decisions.

Young adulthood (approximate age 20-30)

The young adult faces the daunting task of discovering ***intimacy versus isolation***. During this stage, individuals wish to seek companionship and intimacy with a significant other, or avoid relationships and become isolated.

Adulthood (approximate age 30-65)

The adult experiences the need to be productive, known as generativity (i.e. creating products, ideas or children) or to be stagnant. The psychosocial crisis in this stage is ***generativity versus stagnation***.

Mature adulthood (approximate age 65 and beyond)

The mature adult centers on older adults reviewing and making an effort to make sense of their life, reflecting on completed goals or doubts and despair about unreached goals and desires. This stage is known as the battle between ***integrity and despair.***

Figure 9.1
EAP sessions need to be designed with the client's developmental stage and problem solving capability in consideration.

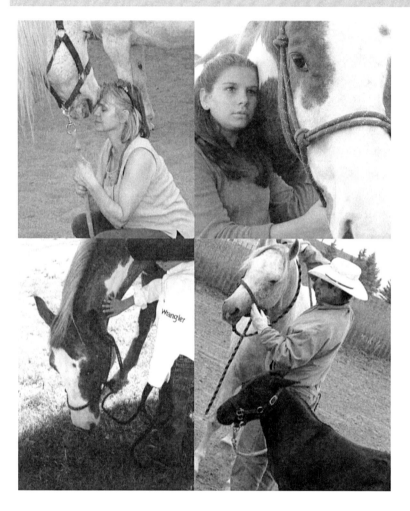

How Age Impacts Equine-Assisted Psychotherapy

Knowing Piaget's and Erikson's stages of development are very helpful in designing and processing EAP activities appropriately for each client. Many EAP professionals argue that Equine-Assisted Psychotherapy, in its truest form, requires a higher awareness of cognition. In order to process and compare the horse activity to life situations, one must be in at least the concrete operational stage of cognitive development. For maximum benefit in processing, the client who is able to think abstractly and transfer this metaphorical scenario to real life is able to leave with an awareness of the generalizability of the lessons learned. However this does not mean that a client of lower cognitive development cannot benefit from EAP.

    For example, one patient I encountered and worked with off and on for two years using EAP was nine years old. She had some learning disabilities and moderately functioning IQ. Due to her level of comprehension and cognitive development, we had to adjust her activities to meet her where she was developmentally. We did little processing other than very black and white, concrete points that were happening in the moment. One day toward the end of her therapy with us, we had seen much growth in her cognitive development and wanted to test her ability to think abstractly. So, I asked her, "In what ways are you like this horse you are working with?" She looked at me and began to laugh. She said, "I'm not like a horse because I don't even like hay!" Although, she later did find some similarities. They both had long red hair and loved to run. It was very apparent that she was developmentally unable to relate the concrete to a hypothetical situation. Nevertheless, by focusing on the concrete, we were able to successfully address her therapeutic issues of trust, low self-esteem, poor communication skills, and poor social skills. In a sense, the EAP activities allowed her to revisit the stages of psychosocial development from infancy and then progress forward. It was obvious she had some unresolved conflicts from the beginning that she needed to work through before she was able to progress on with her development. By the end, she could catch, halter and lead the horse by herself. She even got the horse to follow her over a jump. This testimony is a reminder that it is critical to consider the developmental stage of the client. In Houck, Jung, McKissick, Hamilton, & Lytle (2008), it is consensus that when working with children less verbal processing is needed. Young children learn metaphorically through the experiences they have with the horses, and then use those experiences to resolve conflict outside the arena in other parts of their lives.

    The same question asked of a client in formal operational development will be answered very differently from the child in the pre-operational stage. The more advanced the development the more advanced their ability to verbalize the metaphorical component in the sessions and the more aware they will be of possible life applications while in the arena. A primary reason for this variation depends on the client's level of cognitive development, despite age. For example, when asked, "What did the horses teach you about life?" clients in different developmental stages had the following answers:

> *"Sometimes, like the horses, people need help getting over bad habits."*
> Client, age 12

> *"I learned that fear does not help me when I saw Cody (a therapy horse). What I learned about fear was the more fear you have inside of you, it takes a long time to trust someone. I looked at Cody and saw fear. I have had a time like that the first time I came, it was hard for me not to cry or anything due to my fear of the horses. I was not giving the horse a chance. I did not try. That was fear. I now know that my fear can affect my relationships with other people. That's what also helped me. I hope we can all get rid of our fears by the end of the program."*
> Client, age 14

> *"The horses taught me patience, contentment, and joy in the moment. I had to have these things when I was with the horses because they don't respond if you're not patient with them and fully present. In everyday life, I need to be fully present. My eating disorder took away my life, so that while my body was present (what little was left of it), my spirit was never there. In order to be whom God wants me to be and to experience the joy that He has in store for me, I need to be fully present with Him in each and every day that He blesses me with. In EAP, if my body was there and my mind was not, not only did I miss important points, I also exposed myself to the risk of injury. In my walk with God every day, if I am not fully present with Him, I risk losing out on important points and opportunities, as well as exposing myself to a desolate existence without Him, which is much worse than physical injury."*
> Client, age 23

The variations in development, despite age, are apparent in the previous client responses. This difference in response demonstrates how diverse clients' perceptions of an activity can be. Understanding where the client is developmentally is a vital component in maximizing the benefits of EAP for the client. Otherwise, the processing of an activity may be too complex or too elementary for the participants affecting the depth and amount of valuable information the experience can provide for the client.

In conclusion, it is critical that the treatment team be able to function as a team at the highest level of cognitive functioning, formal operational stage, if they plan on working with clients who potentially could operate in or reach for the formal operational stage of development. This will enable the team to be more flexible in the depth of processing they are able to provide. Robertson and Boyce (2008) summarize to say that horses and humans interact in meaningful ways in EAP sessions. Horses sway over the human psyche of all ages, reinforcing the value of challenging suppositions about learning, self-awareness and safety.

Topics of Discussion:

1. What were the main components of the two developmental theories presented in this chapter? How do they come into play in an EAP session?

2. Do you agree with the argument that a client must have reached the concrete operational stage of development before benefiting from EAP? Give reasons to justify your answer.

3. What level of development do you think the following clients are operating from based on their responses? Give reasons for your answers.

"The horses taught me that you can get respect through fear or through just being a good person. People want to be with you when you are nice to them." Client, age 13

"The horses taught me that everybody needs to follow instructions so you won't be punished."

                                              Client, age 16

"Boundaries are good because they keep the horses safe, keep people safe, help the horses know where to go, and help people know what is expected."

                                                Client, Age 9

"Every horse is different, so you have to change to work with that horse. It's the same way for people."   **Client, age 11**

"The blind-fold activity was most meaningful to me. The activity described my relationship with God. The obstacle course represented my life; and in some ways, I am blindfolded as I go along because I don't know what lies ahead. I have my family beside me to help and insure my safety --- as long as I ask for their help. The person leading the horse represented God – leading me through life. I can only imagine how wild and dangerous it would be without anyone leading the horse in that big pasture. That's what my life would be like without God in control – a WRECK!"

                                                Client, Age 14

4. *Describe the benefit of understanding the psychosocial stages of development for the EAP treatment team? With this knowledge, what might the team do differently when setting up EAP activities?*

5. *What other developmental theories would be beneficial for the EAP treatment team to be aware of? In what ways would this information help?*

Chapter Notes

Chapter Notes

10 WORKING WITH GROUPS

Objectives:
- **Identify pros and cons of group therapy**
- **Explore concerns to consider when forming a group**
- **Identify the various types of groups**
- **Assess working with special populations**
- **Analyze the stages of group development**

While one-on-one counseling sessions may be the best option for some individuals and issues, particularly for those who might pose a danger to themselves or others, group therapy is also a valuable tool for many populations and needs. Group therapy can serve as an adjunct treatment to individual therapy or as the complete treatment plan approach depending on the needs of the client and the abilities of the therapeutic team. In this chapter, we will explore many important components to think about as a treatment team when considering group therapy as the therapy format of choice for EAP client(s). We will discuss the benefits of group therapy, practical considerations when forming a group, various group types, and special populations.

Benefits of Group Therapy

In general, it has been discovered that group therapy is as effective as individual therapy in bringing about change (Sleek, 1995). Group sessions are very useful for developing social skills such as communication and teamwork, which make the group setting ideal for companies and organizations as well as for many clients. For instance, group sessions are particularly beneficial for adolescents as they are so strongly influenced by peer interactions and opinions. Feelings of isolation, abandonment and grief due to divorce, death or serious illness of a loved one are other examples of issues that are often addressed in the group setting.

Group counseling has a number of advantages as a vehicle for helping people make changes in their attitudes, feelings, behaviors, and beliefs about themselves and others. One advantage of group counseling is that participants can explore their styles of relating with others and learn more effective social skills. Another is that members of the group can discuss their perceptions of one another and receive valuable feedback on how they are being perceived in the group. In many ways, the counseling group provides a re-creation of the participants' everyday world, especially if the membership is diverse with respect to age, interests, background, socioeconomic status, and type of problem (Corey, 1995; Kottler & Shepard, 2011).

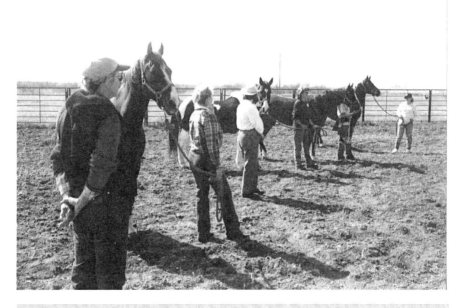

Figure 10.1 – This group just completed an activity and is now checking in.

A well-functioning counseling group offers understanding and support that fosters the members' willingness to explore the problems they have brought to the group. Each individual participant achieves a sense of belonging; and through the cohesion that develops, he/she learns ways to become intimate and caring while challenging one another on issues and behaviors. In a supportive group atmosphere, members can experiment with alternative behaviors. They can practice these behaviors in the group, where they receive encouragement and suggestions on how to apply what they are learning to their experiences in the outside world. They can compare the perceptions they have of themselves with the perceptions others have of them and then decide what to do with this information. In essence, the group gets a glimpse of the kind of people they would like to become, and each individual comes to understand what is preventing him/her from becoming that person (Corey, 1995; Kottler & Shepard, 2011).

Formation of the Group

Therapeutic groups are determined by many factors: age; gender; developmental levels; emotional, mental, or behavioral issues; personality types; and association. Examples of associative groups are families, companies, organizations, clubs, and churches.

The basic criterion for the selection of group members is whether they will contribute to the group or whether they will be counterproductive. Some people can quite literally drain the energy of the group so that little is left for productive work. Also, the presence of certain people can make group cohesion difficult to attain (Corey, 1995; Kottler & Shepard, 2011).

Some questions the treatment team should ask themselves when determining whether group counseling is the appropriate choice:

- Is the individual a physical or emotional danger to self or others?
- Is the individual ready or able to work with others?
- Is the individual trying to address a problem that is social in nature?
- What can group sessions provide for this individual that individual sessions cannot?
- Can the treatment team work with the entire group without compromising or neglecting any of the individuals in the group?

Practical Concerns in the Formation of a Group

When forming a group, there are many factors that the treatment team must consider: open versus closed group, voluntary versus involuntary membership, homogeneous versus heterogeneous groups, group size, frequency and length of meetings, group duration and meeting place. Corey (1995) and Kottler & Shepard (2011) explain each factor which should be considered when the EAP team is determining the format of a group.

Open versus Closed Groups. Whether the group will be open or closed may in part be determined by the population and the setting. There are some distinct advantages to both kinds of groups. In a closed group, no new members are added for the predetermined duration of its life. This practice offers a stability of membership that makes continuity possible and fosters cohesion. A problem with closed groups is that if too many members drop out, the group process is drastically affected. In an open group, new members replace those who are leaving, and this can provide new stimulation. A disadvantage of the open group is that new members may have a difficult time becoming a part of the group, because they are not aware of what has been discussed before they joined. Therefore, if the flow of the group is to be maintained, the leader needs to devote time and attention to preparing new members and helping them become integrated.

Voluntary versus Involuntary Membership. Should groups be composed only of members who are there by their own choice, or can groups function even when they include involuntary members? This is a debate amongst therapists in the EAP field. Obviously, there are a number of advantages to working with a group of clients who are willing to invest themselves in the group process. However, in many agencies and institutions, practitioners are expected to lead groups with an involuntary clientele. It is therefore important for these counselors to learn how to work within such a structure rather than holding on to the position that they can be effective only with a voluntary population. The horses are effective with both populations. By utilizing the horses in the sessions, the practitioner has an added advantage in bringing down the defensive walls of all clients, including clients who may not have chosen to attend.

Homogeneous versus Heterogeneous Groups. Group leaders need to decide the basis for the homogeneity of the groups. **Homogeneous** means to be composed of people who, for example, are similar in ages, such as a group for children, for adolescents, or for the elderly. Other homogeneous groups are those based on a common interest or problems (i.e. Alcoholics Anonymous). While homogeneous membership can be more appropriate for certain target populations with definite needs, heterogeneous membership has some definite advantages for many personal-growth groups. A **heterogeneous** group, by representing a microcosm of the social structure that exists in the everyday world, offers the participants the opportunity to experiment with new behavior, develop social skills, and get feedback from many diverse sources. If a simulation of everyday life is desired, it is helpful to have a range of ages, backgrounds, interests, and concerns.

Group Size. The desirable size for an EAP group depends on factors such as the age of the clients, the type of group, the group experience (i.e. EAP activities planned), the experience of the EAP team, and the types of problems explored. Another element to be taken into consideration is whether the group has two leaders or more; and in all EAP activities, the number of horses used must also be considered. For ongoing EAP groups with adults, eight to ten members with one therapist and horse professional is desirable. EAP groups with children may be as small as three or four. Adolescent groups are at their best with about six to eight members present. In general, the group should have enough people to afford ample interaction so that it doesn't drag and yet be small enough to give everyone a chance to participate frequently without losing the sense of "group." Because the number of horses does increase the total involved in the arena, this factor is very unique to EAP and must also be evaluated. Horses become a part of the group or it could be considered that the group becomes part of the herd. For instance, if a group has eight participants and four horses, the facilitators must consider that now their group has increased to twelve and must be observed as such.

Frequency and Length of Meetings. How often should groups meet? And for how long? These issues also depend on the type of group and, to some extent, on the experience of the leaders. The age of participants should also be a factor in determining how long to meet. With EAP, you must remember that much information and insight is gained in a shorter amount of time. Therefore, if you ask a family or adolescents to work more than three hours in one setting, you may be limiting their comprehension and/or retention of insights gained due to overload of information.

Group Duration. The duration varies from group to group, depending on the type of group and the population. Corey (1995) emphasizes that the group should be long enough to allow for cohesion and productive work yet not so long that it seems to drag on interminably. Brabender & Fallon (2009) believe that any particular time span that is defined up front to the group provides both opportunities and challenges. Groups aware of a distinct time limit, particularly if that time limit is brief as in EAP, have an added pressure to make progress. This pressure can lead the group to be more proactive in tackling work that otherwise might be put off. Once again, EAP is a very intense and intrusive approach to therapy. The treatment goals need to be considered when evaluating the duration of a group.

Meeting Place. Another pre-group concern is the setting. Privacy, a certain degree of attractiveness (professionalism), and a place that allows for face-to-face interaction are crucial. With EAP, these considerations are critical and cannot be jeopardized just the same. The meeting place needs to consider weather conditions as well. For example, you may not want to offer a group during the winter months if you only have an outdoor arena available (depending on your geographical location).

Types of Associative Groups

In addition to the practical factors to consider when forming a group, the EAP team must also determine who the target audience will be and the goals of this group. There are various types of associative groups to be considered.

Families. Within the last 2 decades there has been a dramatic shift in the structure of the traditional American family. This shift has included an increase in divorce, single-parent households, and dual-career families. Demographics on family patterns indicate that between 40% and 50% of all marriages end in divorce, and 80% of all divorced persons remarry within four to five years (Clapp & Rudolph, 1993). An important factor to consider is the ability of families to effectively cope and adapt to the stress associated with these transitions. Divorced, remarried, single-parent, adoptive, and dual-career families experience stresses and strains that can tax a family's ability to cope (Clapp & Rudolph, 1993).

When families are in crisis they experience tension and anxiety, resulting in feelings of disorganization and disequilibration. A crisis places extraordinary demand on a family's standard coping resources (Shank & Kinney, 1987). Families do better if they can unite against outside forces. Painful experiences, if dealt with properly, can sometimes be good lessons. It's not the stress families experience; it's what they do with stress that matters. The optimal range of stress gives families sufficient challenges so that they are energized to grow and develop, but not so much stress that they cannot succeed (Pipher, 1996). Families that cope well experience their world as tough but manageable. With effort, they can be successful and this success brings self-regard. Healthy families know that no experience is worthless if it teaches lessons. Extracting meaning from suffering heals the family (Pipher, 1996).

When families initially encounter strains or stress, often they become self-absorbed. They have a tendency to withdraw from their usual life activities and to experience a loss of control over their lives (Austin, 1998). The family members become so absorbed in their individual problems that they have difficulty functioning as a group. EAP group sessions can be the ideal therapy for such families because it forces the family to re-group to work together instead of as wounded individuals. Once engaged in an interactive therapeutic activity like EAP, families can begin to perceive themselves as being able to successfully interact with their environments, to start to experience feelings of success and mastery, and to take steps toward regaining a sense of control. Such outcomes are empowering. Families come to realize that they are not passive victims but can take action to restore the health of their family (Austin, 1998).

The family setting also promotes accountability, a sense of belonging, as well as the importance of group effort and family accomplishment (Ham et al., 1998). The issues raised and the techniques used to manage the horse's behavior in EAP help teach the families skills needed for their own practical life application. This translates to other areas of therapy, enabling the family to relate more openly (Ham et al., 1998). As a result, EAP helps families to respond proactively rather than reactively as a group.

Most research focuses on what problems exist and how often they occur rather than on the processes families engage in concerning them. Researchers have largely failed to examine factors that help families develop resilience to the stresses of life and relationships. One area of focus in EAP is to examine how encountering and overcoming problems constitutes a resource that contributes to growth in the family members and strengthens family relationships (Wright et al., 1994). In sum, the goals for families participating in EAP include improving stress management skills, building family strengths, and enhancing family communication skills. Therefore, EAP explores ways of helping families effectively balance cohesion and adaptability to mesh with the needs of developing family members.

Business Groups. Business groups are much like family therapy -- a system that functions together to reach a common goal. Therefore, the techniques that are used with families will also greatly benefit a business. Nevertheless, the goals for working with a business may be very different than the family goals. A first step to corporate development is determining the business's objectives and goals for the business and the training. These types of activities build team work, communication, cooperation, and creative thinking; all of which are vital in a business' success and cohesion. With the focus being more on learning, coaching and education, corporate groups are often referred to as **Equine-Assisted Learning (EAL)**. The distinction between EAP and EAL is discussed further in chapter 8.

When an EAL training is effective, participants often return to the workplace with an afterglow. They may seem refreshed and display a renewed enthusiasm. They may enjoy a heightened awareness of old behaviors and new possibilities. They often invite dialogue and talk excitedly about new tools for implementing changes. Then the phone rings, memos land, workday problems set in and – what happens? While operating "out-of-the box" in the EAL session, anything may have seemed possible: cooperation, exploration, playfulness, supportiveness, openness, introspection, risk. Now, back in the box of familiarity, with its demands and priorities, spoken and unspoken expectations, rewards and restrictions, will any of the meaning stick (Smolowe, Butler, Murray, 1999?

Prince (2009) emphasizes that EAL provides incredible insights and metaphors for working through the goals of the corporate group. In Table 10.1, Trinity Counseling Center EAL staff development survey (personal communications, spring 2000) indicates some additional advantages or lessons business participants gained upon completion of an EAP corporate development experience:

Table 10.1 Corporate Training Testimonials

> "Hands on experience created real life challenges immediately."

> "Eye opening to realize that a business can get into the same 'stuck place' as families."

> "Working together as a staff really highlighted some aspects that are true about how we do and do not work together in the office."

> "Characteristics of personalities come out as we were challenged by the horses."

> "Actually seeing the differences, likenesses, obstacles, etc. in a person's life and how that affects work was amazing and helpful."

> "Group and relationship dynamics surfaced so quickly and vividly."

> "Quickly brings to light many of the relationship and work dynamics that a staff experiences on a daily basis."

> "Shows a need to change."

An EAL experience, of course, is only a beginning. It can hold up a mirror to old behaviors, create a forum for exploring new possibilities, and suggest new pathways for navigating corporate waters. But the real work of behavioral change begins after participants emerge from the EAL environment and return to their daily work lives (Smolowe, et. al., 1999).

When a group returns from an EAL experience, they may walk a new walk and talk a new talk—for a while. The question is, once the residual exhilaration and excitement wear off, does anything remain? One of the best gauges of enduring impact is the effort that participants make to translate the learnings into concrete practices (Smolowe, et. al., 1999). Therefore, helping the group translate their insights into action while involved in the EAL experience will help facilitate long term change.

Non-Associative Groups

Children. Counseling groups for children can serve preventive or rehabilitative purposes. Group counseling is often suggested for children who display behaviors or attributes such as excessive fighting, self-image issues, inability to get along with peers, violent outbursts, lack of supervision at home, and neglected appearance. Small groups can provide children with the opportunity to express their feelings about these and the related problems. Identifying children who are developing serious emotional and behavioral problems is extremely important. If these children can receive psychological assistance such as EAP at an early age, they stand a better chance of coping effectively with the developmental tasks they must face later in life (Corey, 1995; Shechtman, 2007). Jennifer Petersen, therapist for a day treatment program (personal communications, July 2013), states, "Many of the children in the foster care system are at a disadvantage when it comes to learning how to make positive life decisions. With EAP, these children learn that they are capable of making decisions and are asked to walk through that process and learn from it."

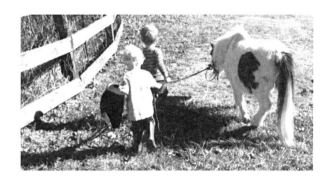

Figure 10.2

Opportunities for growth and learning are tailored to the group's needs and goals.

Adolescents. Corey (1995) and Shechtman (2007) continue to explain how the adolescent years can be extremely lonely ones, and it is not unusual for an adolescent to feel that no one is there to help. Adolescence is also a time of deep concerns and key decisions that can affect the course of one's life. Dependence/independence struggles, acceptance/rejection conflicts, identity crises, search for security, pressures to conform, and the need for approval are all part of this period. Many adolescents are pressured to perform and succeed, and they frequently experience severe stress in meeting these external expectations. Group therapy is especially suited for adolescents because it gives them a place to express conflicting feelings, explore self-doubts, and come to the realization that they share these concerns with their peers. EAP groups allow adolescents to openly question their values and to actively modify those that need to be changed. In the EAP group, adolescents can learn to communicate with their peers, benefit from the modeling provided by the leader, and safely experiment with reality and test their limits. Another unique value of group counseling for adolescents is that it offers them a chance to be instrumental in one another's growth. Because of the opportunities for interaction available in the EAP group situation, the participants can express their concerns and be heard, and they can help one another on the road toward self-understanding and self-acceptance (Corey, 1995; Shechtman, 2007).

Elderly. Counseling groups can be valuable for the elderly in many of the same ways that they are of value to adolescents. As people grow older, they often experience isolation, and many of them, seeing no hope of meaning – let alone excitement – in their future, may resign themselves to a useless life. Like adolescents, the elderly often feel unproductive, unneeded, and unwanted. Another problem is that many older people accept myths about aging, which then become self-fulfilling prophecies. An example is the misconception that elderly people can't change or that once they retire, they will be doomed to depression (Corey, 1995). EAP groups can help older people challenge these myths and deal with the developmental tasks that they, like any other age group, must face in such a way that they can retain their integrity and self-respect. The EAP group situation can assist people in breaking out of their isolation and offer the elderly the encouragement necessary to find meaning in their lives so that they can live fully and not merely exist.

Special Populations – Physical and/or Cognitive Disabilities.
When special populations such as physical and/or cognitive disabilities begin to get addressed in Equine-Assisted Psychotherapy, the line can easily gray between EAP and therapeutic riding. Some EAP professionals believe that EAP in its truest form is most appropriate for a client population who can think abstractly (average age is 10 to 12 years of age in normal development) and is able to safely maneuver without limitations around the horses for ground activities. If a person fits this criteria, no matter what age, then he/she would benefit fully from the EAP experience. Other EAP professionals argue that by the treatment team imposing their own guidelines or beliefs onto a client, they are

limiting what the client is capable of doing. Professionals agree on the fact that the activities need to be developmentally and physically designed to be appropriate for the client. Regardless of the client's mental and/or physical situation, the question remains, "Can EAP work for that client if the client is willing to work for results?" From the standpoint in favor of being nondiscriminatory regarding EAP, the professionals argue that EAP is to mirror their life. These professionals pose a legitimate question, "If the treatment team is putting limits on the client, how is the client ever supposed to discover how to succeed in a world that continually puts limits on them as well?"

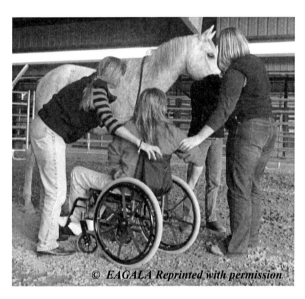

Figure 10.3

This EAP activity is being done with all the client's therapeutic needs being considered. Can EAP be done with someone in a wheelchair? What do you think?

With regard to physical handicaps, safety concerns must be considered by the EAP team and client as in all EAP activities. These issues seem to be magnified when doing ground activities with a client with physical handicaps. Once again, the professionals in the field have varied opinions as to how to handle these situations. Nevertheless, many life lessons can be taught through the struggle of EAP activities seeming more difficult due to their physical impairments. EAP may be exactly what the person needs to find new ways to deal with a world that is not totally "handicap accessible." This situation will require much skill and creativity on the EAP team's part.

Stages of Group Development

Corey (1995) explains that all groups go through a set of phases or stages that are to be expected. Interestingly enough, in EAP these stages seem to be magnified. It is important to expect and understand the stages of group growth and development, as well as, to be aware of the warning signs of getting "stuck" in one stage and not moving on. For group closure to occur successfully, it is important for a group to pass through all stages. A healthy group will have no problems passing through all stages. The key to a healthy group is the group leaders.

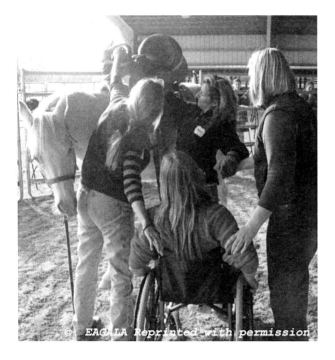

Figure 10.4

Creativity and adaptability on the EAP treatment team's part reduces limitations for all participants.

Pre-Group Considerations – Setting group goals

Ideally, the members decide for themselves the specific goals of the group experience. Corey (1995) describes some of the general goals shared by group members which are also found in EAP groups:

- ➢ to learn to trust oneself and others
- ➢ to achieve self-knowledge and develop a sense of one's unique identity

- to increase self-acceptance, self-confidence, and self-respect in order to achieve a new view of oneself
- to find alternative ways of dealing with normal developmental issues and resolving certain conflicts
- to increase self-direction, autonomy, and responsibility toward oneself and others
- to become aware of one's choices and to make choices wisely
- to make specific plans for changing certain behaviors and to commit oneself to follow through with these plans
- to learn more effective social skills
- to learn how to confront others with care, concern, honesty, and directness
- to clarify one's values and decide whether and how to modify them

Stage 1 – Orientation and Exploration. The early phase of a group is a time for orientation and determining the structure of the group. Once again, Corey (1995) adequately lists some of the distinguishing events of this stage as follows:

- Participants test the atmosphere and get acquainted.
- Members learn the norms and what is expected, learn how the group functions, and learn how to participate in a group.
- Members display socially acceptable behavior, risk taking is relatively low, and exploration is tentative.
- Group cohesion and trust are gradually established if members are willing to express what they are thinking and feeling.
- Members are concerned with whether they are included or excluded, and they are beginning to define their place in the group.
- A central issue is trust versus mistrust.
- There are periods of silence and awkwardness; members may look for direction and wonder what the group is about.
- Members are deciding whom they can trust, how much they will disclose, how safe the group is, whom they like and dislike, and how much to get involved.
- Members are learning the basic attitudes of respect, empathy, acceptance, caring, and responding – all attitudes that facilitate trust building.

Stage 2 – Transition Stage: Dealing with Resistance. Corey (1995) states that the transitional phase of a group's development is marked by feelings of anxiety and defenses in the form of various resistances. At this time members are:

- Wondering what they will think of themselves if they increase their self-awareness and wondering about others' acceptance or rejection of them.
- Testing the leaders, horses, and other members to determine how safe the environment is.
- Struggling with whether to remain on the periphery or to risk getting involved.
- Experiencing some struggle for control and power and some conflict with other members or the leader.
- Learning how to work through conflict and confrontation.
- Feeling reluctant to get fully involved in working on their personal concerns because they are not sure others in the group will care about them.
- Observing the leaders and horses to determine if they are trustworthy and learning from each person how to resolve conflict.
- Learning how to express themselves so that others will listen to them.

Stage 3 – Working Stage: Cohesion and Productivity. Corey (1995) explains that when a group reaches the working stage, the central characteristics include the following:

- The level of trust and cohesion is high.
- Communication within the group is open and involves an accurate expression of what is being experienced.
- Members interact with one another freely and directly.
- There is a willingness to risk threatening material and to make oneself known to others; members bring to the group personal topics they want to discuss and understand better.
- Conflict among members is recognized and dealt with directly and effectively.
- Feedback is given freely and accepted and considered non-defensively.
- Confrontation occurs in a way in which those doing the challenging avoid slapping judgmental labels on others.

- Members are willing to work outside the group to achieve behavioral changes.
- Participants feel supported in their attempts to change and are willing to risk new behavior.
- Members feel hopeful that they can change if they are willing to take action; they do not feel helpless.

Stage 4 – Final Stage: Consolidation and Termination. Corey (1995) concludes that during the final phase of a group the following characteristics are typically evident:

- There may be some sadness and anxiety over the reality of separation.
- Members are likely to pull back and participate in less intense ways, in anticipation of the ending of the group.
- Members are deciding what courses of action they are likely to take.
- There may be some fears of separation as well as fears about being able to implement in daily life some of what was experienced in the group.
- Members may express their fears, hopes, and concerns for one another and tell one another how they were experienced.
- Members may evaluate the group experience.
- There may be talk about follow-up meetings or some plan for accountability so that members will be encouraged to carry out their plans for change.

Groups create many added challenges for an EAP treatment team. Nevertheless, the benefits are astounding. Despite the type of group, the group dynamics in the arena present another opportunity to mirror real life for clients, allowing the EAP treatment team to walk along side them as they grapple with relationships, not only with the horses but with others as well.

Topics for Discussion:

1. Neuroscientists have recently discovered that many people who have language processing disorders, also have difficulty "reading" people, as both skills seem to be located in the prefrontal lobes. How would this discovery affect your choice between traditional talk therapy and EAP? Which do you feel would work best in helping this population address problems with social skills? Explain.

2. *Recent research is demonstrating that many behavioral problems are due to neurological miss-wiring. Could a physiologically-caused behavioral trait be addressed through EAP? If so, how?*

3. *Is group therapy beneficial for all populations and age groups? Explain and give examples.*

4. *There is a dispute among EAP professionals as to the effectiveness of EAP with clients with severe physical or mental disabilities. What is your stance in this debate? Explain.*

Chapter Notes

Chapter Notes

11 PHYSICAL AND EMOTIONAL SAFETY

Objectives:
- **Define aspects of physical and emotional safety**
- **Introduce EAP philosophy to safety**
- **Explore safety considerations with clients and horses**
- **Evaluate setup, equipment, and horses for safety**

Where do people invest their time, energy and money to be safe? The question of what they invest in keeping themselves and others around them safe is their personal philosophy and definition of safety. Without getting into an argument about good vs. bad, or right vs. wrong, the aim of this chapter is to inspire the reader to think, or rethink, their current philosophies on safety (Kersten, March/April, 2003). While general, philosophical approaches to safety will be discussed, this chapter encourages the readers to evaluate their own beliefs about safety and how those beliefs may affect clients' progress.

Safety is one of the most important concerns in all Equine-Assisted Psychotherapy activities. Safety not only protects the EAP team and clients from injury but also teaches a valuable metaphorical lesson about personal safety in the client's life. Do they do a good job of that or not? In many cases, the answer is "no" and it becomes a therapeutic goal to learn a healthier and safer way to approach life.

The simple thought of safety conjures up thoughts of teachers, talking, classes, equipment, and the feeling that it pertains only to horse activities. Safety is very much a part of our life -- safety with horses, cars, school, household items, and much more (Kersten, October 1999).

A majority of the clients in EAP have issues with being safe. Many times, they are victims or victimizers. Either way, they benefit from lessons, education and an understanding of safety. EAP sessions lend themselves to these lessons. Every element of safety that comes up in a session can be therapeutic for the clients, from the time they walk through the door until they leave. As the safety issues arise and are remedied, the EAP team can easily draw parallels to the client's life and how that client keeps him/herself safe in different situations at home, school, or work. (Kersten, October 1999).

The primary concern for any program or practice is safety. In this model, realistic safety is promoted, looking at both the physical and emotional safety (EAGALA, 2012). In this chapter, we will focus on ensuring the physical and emotional safety of clients and horses. This chapter will discuss ways to make facilities safer physically and emotionally. It will also explore topics that are critical for the treatment team to be knowledgeable about to ensure safety. Most importantly, this chapter will take a look at how to ensure that the treatment team is safe and more emotionally secure in handling safety issues.

Physical Safety

Many follow the teaching that one must have lengthy, lecturing safety policies and rules, in order to learn to stay safe. Many EAP professionals challenge that philosophy and actually will say that a focus on having abundant "do not's" as a safety policy is probably less safe. The approach of these professionals is a hands on approach to safety involving observation and knowledge skills versus reacting to everything in fear.

Safety with Clients

Every EAP treatment team should think of their clients while planning activities, taking note of potential dangers and discussing outlet options to avoid injuries. It is assumed that as professionals, the EAP team must know their clients and horses best and should recommend any safety equipment you feel necessary. Many of the EAP training organizations, do not make any safety equipment mandatory; however, safety training is mandatory. Kersten and Thomas (1999) state that simple reliance on any type of safety equipment promotes a false sense of security and diminishes efforts of common sense when developing true safety procedures. Kersten and Thomas (1999) use the following analogy to defend this philosophy: would anyone recommend that a woman go back into a physically abusive relationship and suggest that her solution is to just wear pads and a helmet? Of course not! Others would work to teach the woman how to stay safe. There are two sides to this issue, and EAP professionals are given the choice to decide what works best for clients in various EAP programs.

Likewise, EAP does not promote scaring clients into safety. Telling scary stories (my brother's friend's daughter almost got killed by a horse…), horrible things that can happen to the clients if they don't follow the rules, or sharing scary, traumatic helmet videos can be manipulative and counterproductive. If the EAP team can't enforce guidelines or rules without scare tactics, they may want to explore what that is about. EAP professionals don't want the clients to approach horses or life with fear, but with observation and response skills. If the EAP team responds to situations in fear, the situation is most likely to turn for the worse (EAGALA, 2006).

According to EAGALA (2012), the results of these tactics include the clients becoming so focused on fear that they have difficulty thinking of anything else or being themselves which is an important prerequisite in this model. Additionally, in more immediate crisis situations, this fear causes panic and over-reaction – the two primary reasons people around horses end up getting hurt (EAGALA, 2012).

Safety is not a one-time lesson; it is an ongoing process. There are no safety classes, training lessons, or pieces of equipment that will guarantee anyone's safety. EAP takes safety very seriously, and because of that, the EAP team must continually review their techniques and responses (EAGALA, 2012). EAP encourages the treatment team to question everything and look through realistic lens. This includes the EAP team questioning themselves. Where do the facilitators' fears come from? What are they really about? For example, as a facilitator, do he/she have personal fears of being sued, losing your business, or looking incompetent? EAGALA (2012) emphasizes that EAP professionals must investigate their own transference issues/fears because these issues do affect sessions and focus.

As a result, all EAP professional need to look at their personal approach to safety. They need to consider the emotional effects and potential life lessons/metaphors presented when scary stories are used to control behavior in clients. Does the team want to role model using fear and intimidation as acceptable tools to motivate others? Whatever safety philosophy the team decide upon for their EAP sessions, emotional consequences on the overall safety of your client must also be considered.

Safety with Horses

The following section is about safety around the horse. This information is basic safety that every EAP horse professional should know. This knowledge is not always necessary for the client to know up front. Remember, EAP is not horsemanship for clients. Nevertheless, the horse professional should be a skilled horse person. Just because the treatment team doesn't disclose to the client all the potentially hazardous situations in a session, does not mean that this awareness is not necessary for the treatment team to consider or that the team shouldn't be capable of safety interventions.

Kersten & Thomas (1999) promote that a horse professional's safety knowledge must consider the horse's physical make-up and skeletal structure for the following reasons:

➢ The skeletal make-up – recognize the sharp or protruding bones that could come in contact with the human body.
➢ The more common or normal movements of the horse. This helps the equine professional consider a safety plan without clients coming into harmful contact with the horse.

Kersten & Thomas (1999) report that the majority of accidents which occur involve injuries to the head, hands, and feet. These injuries occur because people are not fully aware of a horse's normal reaction or movement while haltering, grooming and leading. Keeping in mind, horses usually move away from pressure. This means they will normally move away from your body. The exception to this rule is when the horse is spooked or frightened and is attempting to flee. The client can be stepped on or run over when there is opposing or threatening pressure. One important aspect to remember is that the more tools and equipment used, the higher the risk of unsafe situations to arise. It is recommended in EAP to be creative with equipment but be mindful of the risks. The more equipment, the more need for instruction. The more instruction, the closer the session becomes to horsemanship rather than EAP. EAP is about the clients exploring their own solutions to the challenges before them. Many professionals in this field recommend starting with very minimal equipment/props to assess the client's safety situation. Then, as the sessions progress, more opportunities to explore their safety on a more complex level is provided by adding props and equipment. If the client demonstrates that they are not ready to be put in a more complex situation safely, then it is not therapeutically to their advantage to progress there. This is a way of balancing physical and emotional safety.

Leading. If a treatment team chooses to include a halter and lead rope as equipment in an activity, the safety of adding this equipment must be considered prior to the session as well as during the session. Once a horse has been caught and haltered in a session, leading is a common transition. The majority of horse professionals have been educated in various ways to handle a horse. However, even the best handlers are guilty of becoming relaxed and lazy in leading familiar horses. In addition, when the client turns a horse toward him/her, the client is bringing the horse's head and feet closer to his/her head and feet. Kersten & Thomas (1999) remind EAP professionals that they are role models to their clients; they need to practice safety themselves. For example, when horses are being led in and/or taken back to their pen by the equine specialists, they must be aware that their actions may be providing lessons to the client –whether positive or negative.

EAP is not about learning to lead a horse properly; however, it is about the possible life lessons that can be gained by how the client chooses to lead the horse. Is the client's approach to leading one that considers his/her personal safety? Before judging, the horse professional needs to be watching the horse for cues and responses. How the horse responds to the approach is valuable information regarding safety. If the treatment team feels uncomfortable with how the client is maneuvering the lead rope, there are creative options to create a more physically safe environment for the client without jeopardizing emotional safety. These creative solutions also help the session from turning into a horsemanship lesson. For example, if you have a client that continues to twist the lead rope around his/her arm, the first step might be to ask about it. Ask if there is anything in his/her life that they are getting all wrapped up in? If the equine specialist feels that the horse is showing signs and/or situation around the arena indicates that the horse may choose to move quickly away from the client, the treatment team might ask the client to unclip the lead rope and bring it with him/her to come check in. This would be a great time to ask about the client's awareness about getting wrapped up in something that ends up hurting and further exploring how that might look in the client's life. In the next session, an option would be to change from the lead rope to ribbon, twine, marking tape, or some other means to connect to the horse that would break without hurting the client if the horse chose to move away quickly. This option leads to many potential metaphorical opportunities with a reduced physical safety risk. Overall, the treatment team needs to consider the potential benefits verses risks in each leading situation and determine what is in the client's best interest for that session.

Tying. Prior to grooming, most horse professionals and stables have specific areas for tying or securing a horse. This is a very common practice, and hitching posts or crossties are usually supplied. This grooming ritual becomes so routine for horse professionals that it may be done without much thought. However, for EAP, the equine specialist must consider the rules around tying horses in the facility of use. Any time a horse is tied up, the safety risk increases again. Thus, the need to instruct on the importance of using slip knots, having secure hitching post, etc. Once again, in this approach to therapy, less instruction is better. The treatment team must weigh the pros and cons of instruction in this situation considering the potential life lessons. Another option would be to ground tie. It takes additional time and practice but teaches a very good lesson. In fact, ground tying makes a great therapy session especially when dealing with issues of respect and assertiveness. It also eliminates safety concerns centered around tying a horse up. However, if not executed well, you may have to deal with a loose horse. So, where the session takes place also must be considered.

If you determine that a tying activity best meets the treatment goals then proceed with both physical and emotional safety in mind. When securing a horse with a lead rope, it is recommended that it be tied to the highest, most secure object. If the hitching post or tie area is not secure, it moves slightly or makes noise; this too may cause the horse to pull back. The higher the area, the less opportunity the horse has to use its strong front end to inflict damage. Keep in mind the horse should be tied with some sort of safety or quick release knot. The horse could and may pull back at any stage of the grooming process. If the horse pulls back, he may figure out that he is able to get free. However, if he continues to struggle, simply untying him prevents the chance of potentially hazardous problems. It is important to remember, that when a horse pulls back, new handlers will tend to run away, or pull back themselves. This only reinforces the horse's flight response (Kersten & Thomas, 1999). The last instructions need to be to move toward the horse and release the tie. This teaches lessons in crisis intervention while calming the horse and client with a plan of action rather than running from the problem.

Grooming. At any stage, a grooming activity may be deemed therapeutically beneficial. Grooming usually entails close work around the horse's head, legs and body. It occasionally takes longer for some to become accustomed to this task than others, and the horse can become bored, nervous or anxious about being away from the herd. Ground tying while grooming is another great EAP activity. This promotes respect, boundaries, and relationship. Grooming time is a great segue if the treatment team needs a little time to set up another activity. It is also relaxing for many clients; therefore, grooming while processing difficult topics helps some clients communicate more at ease.

Figure 11.1
Grooming a horse has many advantages and metaphorical lessons.

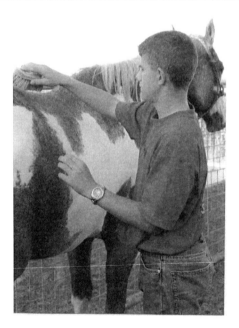

Cleaning Hooves. Kersten & Thomas (2004) state that there are only two things they have found negatively impacting for a horse through the EAP work. One is picking feet and the other is riding.

However, cleaning hooves can lend itself to very powerful metaphorical lessons if handled with therapeutic care. Kersten & Thomas (2004) do not promote picking feet as an activity appropriate for all clients, because it is instructional in nature. So, if the treatment team feels that cleaning hooves is important to the treatment plan, both team members must be aware that it will take more instruction to ensure safety of the horse and they must agree that the teaching moment and lack of self-exploration is more beneficial to the progress for this session. Issues that come up while picking hooves include breaking larger goals into smaller steps, learning to ask different kinds of questions to get different results, building confidence, being mentally and physically capable to support others, trust, working as a team, listening to body language, confronting fear, taking care of yourself, and more (Kersten & Thomas, 2004).

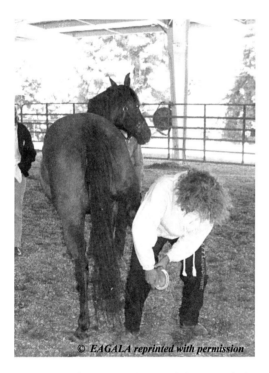

Figure 11.2
Picking the back hoof takes much trust from both the client and the horse.

Having new clients pick up and clean out the horse's hooves can be frightening and rightfully so. Toes being stepped on are probably the most common injury. These injuries usually are not severe but will definitely change the session's focus and may impact responses in sessions to come. The human's feet and legs are slightly diagonal from the horse with feet together. The client's shoulder rests on the horse. Hind legs are different; there is more focus on kicking rather than being stepped on. The front of the horse is heavy and rarely strikes. The rear end is lighter, so is used for kicking. Here it is important to pick up the rear leg and stretch it out to a comfortable position for the horse. Stretch it far enough so that the horse would sooner pull the leg back to his body than leverage to kick. When a horse pulls his leg back to his body, the client is able to move out of danger. Again, actual training in this area as well as practice is highly recommended for all equine specialists (Kersten & Thomas, 1999).

Throughout all EAP activities, the attempt is to provide respect and awareness of safety concerns and to promote common sense thinking rather than scaring the client into reacting fearfully (Kersten & Thomas, 1999). Whether considering leading, tying, grooming, or cleaning hooves, this approach emphasizes weighing the therapeutic benefits versus safety risks and considering the opportunities for metaphorical learning. EAP is about creative problem-solving for the treatment team as well. So, thinking creatively about safety. Overall, EAP is providing experiential lessons exploring clients' personal safety in a physically and emotionally safe environment.

Safety on the Horse

Kersten & Thomas (1999) report that injuries to humans tend to be more serious when the handler becomes the rider. Riding accidents are 75% human error, errors in judgment, equipment, improper training, as well as abilities of the rider and horse. This is one of the main reasons many EAP and training programs recommend 100% groundwork. It is important to remember that the clients served in EAP are most often unprepared for adding more physical and/or emotional risk. EAGALA (2012) states that it is common for facilitators to have a strong desire to put clients on horseback. They encourage teams to investigate this further. They state that groundwork is safer and have found it to be even richer therapeutically. With mounted work comes an increased need for instruction. Anytime instruction is added, the focus shifts away from the client finding answers through exploration and problem-solving into lecturing or teaching.

EAGALA (2012) lists typical reasons facilitators move clients to mounted work:

> - It is the comfort zone of the horse specialist and what he/she is used to doing.
> - It is easier to facilitate a session when clients are on horseback. On the ground, sessions are more challenging to facilitate and take control away from the facilitators. This requires more trust in the horses and clients.
> - The clients want to ride and the facilitator enjoys seeing the client happy.

Some believe that the riding is based on self-imposed limitations placed on ground work possibilities. This can easily happen if the treatment team views this work through horsemanship class lenses. EAGALA (2012) encourages professionals to get out of the box and think more creatively about how the horses can help tell the client's story and provide opportunities for new awarenesses.

In regard to mounted work, the different training institutions and organizations have different standards regarding their guidelines to EAP. In summary, mounted work is no different than any other safety risk taken in session. Again, the treatment team needs to consider the benefits versus risks and remember that some guidelines within their organizational affiliations may influence their decision as well.

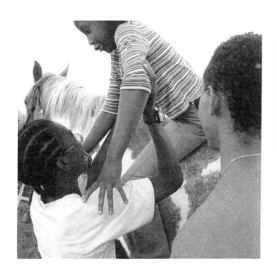

Figure 11.3

Mounted activities rarely use saddles. Saddles can become a crutch or false sense of security.

In the majority of mounted EAP activities, saddles are rarely used as depicted in Figure 11.3. Saddles are designed for accomplishing work, so as long as the client is not roping, fixing, pulling or transporting over long distances, they will ride bareback. Starting the rider out bareback proves to be more effective and safer down the road. Kersten & Thomas (1999) believe that clients that learn to ride bareback first learn better centering and focusing skills, to help them remain balanced and safe. Less emphasis is put on the saddle as a means for safety. The clients then learn to take care of themselves as opposed to relying on the saddle as a crutch. Many metaphors can be found in bareback riding when a client reaches more advanced therapy. Nevertheless, it is debated among EAP professionals as to the necessity of getting a client on the back of a horse at any point in therapy. Many argue that the same lessons can be communicated through ground activities without risking heightened physical or emotional safety issues.

When riding bareback or in the saddle, clients learn that it is their mental and physical positions that keep them healthy. As activities during bareback riding become more difficult, there may be times when the client becomes unbalanced and may need a safety outlet. Because the clients have no manufactured equipment to assist, they are taught a very specific dismount procedure. The EAP treatment team does not want the client to simply jump off and/or let go. The emergency dismount must be taught and practiced. (Kersten & Thomas, 1999)

This dismount does not work if clients are in the saddle. The clients' feet and clothes can catch on the saddle, dragging them in their attempt to dismount. These techniques need to be practiced in all areas of riding, in arenas, pastures and trails, at all levels of rider ability (Kersten & Thomas, 1999). This emergency dismount, just as all other EAP activities, can be metaphorical for life. This technique teaches clientd that when they feels unsafe or off balance, it is okay to have an exit plan or plan to slow down. This plan must be practiced and defined, just as the emergency dismount is. Clients must identify situations when this plan might need to be implemented in their life. For instance, a client who has been in drug rehab for the last three months and is about to be discharged needs to have a slip-prevention plan, or emergency dismount, before leaving treatment. Life can be "quite a ride" and the client could end up getting "thrown" from his/her path getting hurt there isn't some sort of escape plan or prevention dismount in place.

Nevertheless, most EAP programs support EAGALA (2012) when they express the philosophy of focusing exclusively on ground activities. These ground activities are creative and designed to bring out various mental/emotional health issues. It doesn't matter if the clients are an experienced horse person or not, their issues will come out. EAGALA (2006) finds the groundwork to provide much more mileage therapeutically with clients than when they get on the horse's back. With creative facilitation, the same emergency plan can be explored without adding risks and instruction that comes with riding.

Weather Considerations

Always take weather considerations into account and be aware of hazards associated with them. Horse professionals should be alert to changes in horse behavior and horse needs as weather conditions change. Also, mud or snow can be very slick for clients and/or horses, so take appropriate precautions when working in such conditions.

Cold weather can be a potential safety concern. Just as Kersten (November 1999) states, it is critical for the EAP horse professional to be concerned with the equine partners. They need to be healthy in order to perform as EAP assistants. Horses naturally will adapt to this time of year with additional hair coat and fat layer beneath the skin.

Many times the cold weather reduces time spent with the animals. Even though that may occur, the horse professional still needs to keep up adequate feeding, water and hoof care. It is the equine specialists' job to know their equine partners, so spending adequate time with them even in the cold months is vital to consistently knowing their physical and mental state.

If the EAP team brings clients to the EAP facility throughout the winter, take note of areas of concerns. Keep walkways free from snow. Remember the "t" in safety and look over head, side to side, and on the ground. Again, look for items that may cause injury to the humans and horse. This technique is discussed in more detail in Chapter 12.

During winter sessions, the treatment team must consider all weather related conditions and adapt the session accordingly. For instance, taking breaks and processing in heated areas so clients can warm up might be needed if the clients are so cold they cannot talk without teeth chattering. Also, provide water or warm drinks. If clients get too cold, they may lose focus and become careless in the session (Kersten, November 1999). On the flip side, the treatment team must take note that the horses and clients will respond differently in excessive heat. The time of session and/or location of session may need to be adjusted to avoid the heat of the day and direct sun. In addition, the client's medications may have side effects due to excessive heat; so the mental health professional needs to be aware of any medications the client is taking. As with people, horses get lethargic and docile when really hot. So, this reality needs to be taken into consideration. Weather extremes are natural and out-of-our control; therefore, be aware of their presence but don't be shut down by them. The EAP team must weigh potential benefit versus risk. These situations are potential life lessons – life is unpredictable. How does the client handle it "when the heat is on?" Overall, these are opportunities to observe how well the client takes care of him/herself. Are they prepared for the heat or cold? If not, this could be a therapeutic discussion in regards to their lack of preparation in their life?

Gates

Gates have led to many a problem on ranches, farms and stables. These problems range from being left open to improper hanging or securing of gates and latches. These problems, caused by human error, can lead to incidents and accidents. Always keep this in mind when you do your safety checks on your facility.

Kersten (August 1999) promotes considering safety regarding gates from a physical as well as emotional safety stance. Besides some of the physical safety concerns of gate, it is important to plan in advance how to use the gates to promote emotional safety for the clients. Gates are most known for keeping livestock in. However, it is important to remember a dual purpose of keeping other livestock out.

Livestock may also include humans. It can be simple innocent passersby, or other boarders at the stables. Sometimes, it is the next client showing up for their session. Whatever the case, keep gates closed and latched. Many times, if they are coming in to the arena area, the EAP team may hear the gate being opened and can politely ask them to wait until the current session is finished.

In addition to closing and latching gates, the EAP team may want to implement signs that say simply, "In session" or add also "Please do not disturb." Both horse and clinical professionals may also want to sit down and go over their particular policy with new clients. This policy should include appropriate times and procedures for arriving for sessions at the stable.

It is also advised to instruct clients never to just drop in to visit. Many times, clients, especially younger clients, like to do this when they are feeling down or upset. The treatment team may simply ask that they call prior to coming and set up something after talking. Interruptions like this can be very disruptive to someone else's session. Not only does it take the teams' focus off the client, but also it takes the client's focus off the session. By planning in advance and setting up these guidelines for sessions, the EAP team will be creating a safer environment, physically and emotionally (Kersten, August 1999).

Now, for the metaphorical value, gates can have meaning in sessions. If clients are taking their horse from one space to another as part of the session, the treatment team needs to think twice about the automatic response of shutting the gate for the client. By not doing it for them (if they don't ask), can once again provide an opportunity for learning. For instance, we were working with a group from a local drug rehab. Their task was to get two horses from the big pasture into the round pen. The group got the horses out of the big pasture. The horses took off running when they got to the gate of the round pen. Because the group had not shut the gate to the big pasture, they ran back into the pasture. In discussion, the group shared that it was just like getting them to treatment. They wanted to go back to their old life and because they didn't shut the gate to the old life, they were able to go right back. So, the gate was the lesson for the day. I left them with the question, "What gates in your life need shut?" Remember, everything that happens while your client is in session has potential to be a learning moment.

Other Safety Considerations

Make sure participants are appropriately dressed and let them know what to wear before coming. For example, sandals and other open-toed shoes are not recommended for many safety reasons. Be aware of medications that clients are on which may affect balance or ability to react, as well as sensitivity to light or to overheating.

Kersten & Thomas (1999) remind EAP professionals that all safety discussions within themselves can be good therapy sessions for individuals as well as for families or groups (Kersten & Thomas, 1999). It is important to keep accurate notes of the client's performance of these safety techniques during your session. Compare their performance and handling of safety matters before therapy and during treatment. Kersten (October, 1999) has found that often times, they relate to one another.

With accurate notes and discussion of safety, your last few sessions can be devoted to the clients' safety plan away from therapy, and how they will personally keep themselves safe. For instance, I had a client arrive at her first session in flip flops. She made no eye contact except to say that she loves horses. We were faced with a safety dilemma – Do we let her interact with the horses in flip flops or not? Knowing only that she had just been released from inpatient having attempted suicide, I knew her emotional state was fragile. We weighed our options and decided to let her be a part of this decision. After a discussion about personal safety, she chose to carry on and go catch and halter a horse in her flip flops. Forty-five minutes later, she caught a horse, and we began processing. While in deep conversation, the client's toe got stepped on. The client never acknowledged it or even flinched. She carried on in her explanations. I stopped her and asked what just happened. She said, "The horse stepped on my foot." I pointed out that she gave no signals to the horse or us that she was being hurt. I then asked her if she ever did that in life? She replied, "All the time." She continued to process this safety issue by disclosing, for the first time, that she had recently been raped. Clearly, this is more real and visual for clients to relate to. Numerous metaphors can be applied to making safety an active part of treatment and life (Kersten, October 1999).

Emotional Safety

A primary concern for any EAP program or practice is safety. EAGALA (2012), has a safety philosophy that promotes safety realistically and focuses on the often neglected emotional aspect of safety known as **emotional safety**.

Much of what people around horses have been taught focuses on physical safety. Emotional safety and the emotional well-being of the client are often overlooked. In fact, Kersten & Thomas (2004) report that the old-fashioned "teaching safety" is in itself emotionally damaging to many clients. EAP professionals must operate under a safety approach that never uses scary stories to control behavior in clients. Not only do you not want to role model using fear and intimidation as acceptable tools to motivate others, the emotional consequences of this placed fear actually diminishes safety (Kersten & Thomas, 2004).

Kersten & Thomas (2004) promote that EAP professionals use an approach to safety that involves a more "natural" approach. Since EAP is experiential learning, EAP professionals should address safety situations as they occur. This is helpful therapeutically since it allows the EAP team to observe the clients' true selves rather than their responses to lectures. EAP professionals will begin to see this as a more effective and impactful approach to safety. When the EAP treatment team sees their client begin to place him/herself in a dangerous position, they should never scream, over-react, or run over to protect the client. Think of the reaction of someone when you scream in a panic, "Watch out!" The client will most likely tense up, freeze, and then look in your direction instead of focusing on the horses which is where he/she needs to be watching. Instead, the EAP treatment team observes first. Many times, clients recognize that they have gotten themselves in a precarious situation and remedy it themselves. This even occurs in clients who know nothing about horses. This is important information about the client. Nevertheless, if the EAP treatment team does feel the need to intervene, they should respond, "Johnny, could you come here for a minute?" as they begin to walk calmly towards the client. This results in the client walking towards the team, and consequently, out of the dangerous situation. The team can then use the opportunity as a learning experience through the art of asking questions (Kersten & Thomas, 2004). For instance, "Johnny, what did you see the horses do just then? What do you think that might mean? What were you doing in relationship to them?" Many times, if the client did not see what the horses were doing, the treatment team will send him/her back out there and ask him/her to do the same thing, but this time pay close attention to the horses, and then take the opportunity to ask questions again. Rather than the "lecturing to control behavior" approach, this technique has the benefits of keeping the clients and horses calm and objective, using safety as a great life learning opportunity, placing responsibility on the client, and teaching the most effective safety tool -- observation skills (Kersten & Thomas, 2004).

This is probably one of the most difficult parts of facilitating EAP. Certainly, when first beginning this work, the EAP professional may still employ some lecture and step in and intervene much more frequently. But, as he/she practices doing this work and starts to recognize the benefits of teaching safety through the more natural, experiential approach of using questions, he/she will become more comfortable taking a step back (EAGALA, 2012).

No Lecturing

We have all probably thought or felt that safety training is boring or dull at one time or another. Kersten (February 2000) remembers working for large corporations and even the military where safety training was sitting in front of a T.V. monitor in a classroom watching some boring person describing safety procedures. How many people after flying in airplanes a few times still listen to the airline personnel describe safety procedures in case of an emergency or read the pamphlets in front of them?

People have been conditioned to believe safety is BORING. Webster's dictionary defines "boring" as "tedious or tiresome." When humans take part in tedious or tiresome activities, they become careless and they take short cuts to get the activity over with. This attitude creates in and of itself an unsafe situation (Kersten, February 2000).

Safety is fundamental in life and therapy sessions. It should be thought of as a basic principle to all sessions. Because of its great importance, safety needs to be thought of differently. Remember, every safety issue that arises can be made into therapy sessions and acted out to demonstrate the importance of mental and physical involvement in the clients taking care of themselves.

Rewards

It is very important to teach and model the role that rewards play in safety. People give presents, treats, and rewards for many reasons. When it comes to horses or other animals, people give treats to "help build relationships" or "to feel less guilty." Some professionals may argue that, but Kersten (January 2000) would like to challenge these professionals to really analyze why they may give a horse treats.

Because clients and/or professionals feel they can't communicate well with horses, and they want that loving relationship, they reach for something basic. They reach for something that they know the horse would love, like a treat. Parents sometimes do the same thing when dealing with children – they give a treat to influence behavior and attempt to influence attitudes and feelings. The thinking here is that the horse or child loves this treat; and when I give them this treat, the horse or child then loves me.

Sometimes horse professionals and/or clients may feel guilty about keeping the horses penned up, not seeing them enough, or because they "ride" them. They then give treats prior, during and after a ride or a session. Again, the comparison can be made when considering how parents will deal with children, especially in divorced situations or when both parents work.

Basically, these treats are really for the client or professional himself! This makes them *feel* better (Kohn, 1999) It is recommended that all EAP professionals do some self-examination as to why you may give treats to a horse. This is also another issue to discuss with clients as to why they have such strong desire to give treats. What is that about for them?

With reference to a client's physical and emotional safety, a bribe, treat or reward becomes a regular cost of doing business. With horses, this becomes a normal payment possibly because of our rush to a relationship or because of guilt. Remember that we are discussing EAP as a therapeutic intervention. This chapter is not about training techniques in any way. This philosophy is in no way opposing the use of treats as an operant conditioning tool in animal training. This is therapy, not horsemanship or horse training. The approaches are very different. The thinking behind the use of any outside means to get a desired response must be examined. Is it a "crutch" for the client and/or does it create a safety or boundaries issue?

No matter what your position is on treating horses, EAP professionals need to honestly assess why they may be giving treats to their horses. They need to see if their needs being fulfilled in this way may also be affecting how they deal with their clients, co-workers, or families (Kersten, January 2000).

Fear

Kersten (March/April 2003) argues that society today, through media outlets (news, movies, books, etc.) has conditioned customers to believe that they are incapable of protecting themselves, that they do not possess the ability or know how to keep themselves safe. Through such media and marketing companies, people are being trained to prepare for victimization and told they are powerless. EAP professionals need to challenge this false belief within their client's belief system. In fact, the safety philosophy for EAP squarely opposes it.

"Ad-fear-tising," as De Becker (2002) calls it, is exactly what drives the multi-billion dollar safety market. Nothing in this world gets the attention of people and animals as reliably as fear. Or, as Edmund Burke said it, "No passion so effectually robs the mind of all its powers of acting and reasoning as fear" (Kersten, March/April 2003). Fear is a moneymaker; it also is falsely used to promote artificial experts. People all over the world claim "expert status" in a field by pointing out the dangerous side of routine objects and experiences. If their arguments are not convincing, they are usually able to support their claims with a scary story, propagating fear in order to sell you their product or service, as well as the idea that you are indeed helpless. The motivation of those who sell scary stories is always rooted in personal gain.

It is necessary to investigate further the fear reaction, motive, and response to better understand safety and security in a realistic, sensible manner. Fear can be broken down into true fear and unwarranted fear. True fear is the response to being in the presence of real danger. Unwarranted fear is the reaction to a memory or image of perceived fear. Useless safety precautions are based upon imagine threats or concerns, which are not truly happening at the present. Those who are motivated by fear, however, attempt to make reality match imagination through stories or threats. If they don't succeed in scaring you into their fear-based belief system, they may turn coats and actually wish harm upon you to prove their point. Kersten (March/April 2003) promotes that "safety-minded" and vengeful should be mutually exclusive characteristics.

Threats and scare tactics are seldom issued from a position of power. Fear- based people use the word "could" frequently. Take a closer look at any, "Could this happen . . .?" question. The answer to a "could" question is always "yes." A better question might be, "Will this happen...?" or "Will this always happen...?" to realistically evaluate situations.

When clients' focus, time, and energy are spent on unrealistic fears, they may miss the genuine safety concerns in our midst. In EAP sessions, is the treatment team teaching the clients to be powerless and superstitious, or do they allow them to learn through their own problem-solving experiences (Kersten, March/April 2003)?

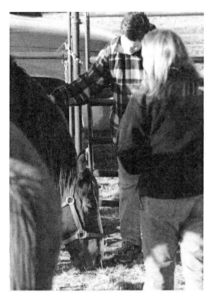
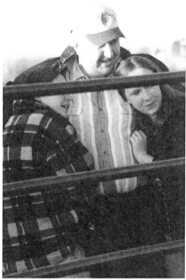

Figure 11.4 Emotional Safety
Family therapy can be challenging but often brings down walls which result in family closeness.

Every animal on earth has an innate system to warn off danger, despite the occasional enjoyment of risk and its accompanying adrenaline. The human alert system is very efficient, and works best when it is accurately informed. Through observation, knowledge, and proper response, we handle risky, frightening and dangerous situations.

Like a muscle, a client's alert system becomes stronger with use. Like any skill, it is possible to forget how to best use this alert system. According to Kersten (March/April 2003) if you should read about, interview, or work with professional soldiers, athletes, or the like, they will tell you that the greatest enemy in any dangerous situation is panic. Reactions to fear and danger vary on an individual basis, still each individual benefits from using a natural, well-informed response.

All EAP activities provide ample opportunity to investigate a client's survival system and responses to fear and risk. For this reason, EAP treatment team members are better served by un-training themselves from automatic alarm and stunned reactions. These irrational reactions shut off realistic perceptions, stymie creativity, and prevent alternative options from forming a more positive outcome. When the EAP treatment team stops thinking and reacts physically, they tend to focus on an imaginary perception of the worst-case scenario as though it were really occurring.

Overall, the EAP treatment team must remember that safety is never about a one-time lesson; it is an ongoing process. There is no class, training lesson, or piece of equipment that will guarantee anyone's safety. EAP professionals need to take safety very seriously, and because of that, continually investigate things thoroughly. Question everything and look through a realistic lens. Additionally, question yourself. Where do your fears come from? What are they really about? (i.e. getting sued, losing your business, looking incompetent, etc.) All EAP professionals must investigate their own transference issues on the horses because these issues do affect the sessions (Kersten & Thomas, 2004).

Topics for Discussion:

1. *Distinguish the difference between physical and emotional safety. Give an example of a safety scenario and discuss how to address the issue considering both physical and emotional safety.*

2. *Describe two different safety scenarios other than the examples in this chapter including specific safety issues or dilemmas. Discuss the life lessons/metaphors about personal safety that could be drawn from such instances.*

3. *There are many debates amongst EAP professionals that revolve around safety. Discuss your view on helmets and mounted activities in an EAP session?*

4. *In addition to the above debates, the argument continues within the field as to whether safety lectures should be given at the introduction of all EAP sessions or not. What are your thoughts about safety only being brought up as it becomes an issue?*

Chapter Notes

CHAPTER 11

Chapter Notes

12 SETTING UP A SESSION

Objectives:
- **Explore procedure for setting up a safe work area**
- **Define the tools and equipment needed for facilitation**
- **Discuss criteria for horse selection and the impact variety has on session outcome**
- **Outline basic criteria to consider when designing an EAP activity**

One of the many lessons clients and participants get out of Equine Assisted Activities is creativity. Kersten (1999, July) suggests that facilitating EAP helps the treatment team become more creative as well. Sometimes creative thinking gets started with one person and then others add to it. This then creates a rapid pursuit of new ideas. Many times, these ideas will not be thought out very well and safety takes the back seat to simply the achievement of the goal. Kersten (1999, July) reports this to be true in over 50% of the sessions he has conducted. With this in mind, it is very important to examine how to set up an EAP activity to be as safe as possible without hindering the creativity process.

In this chapter, you are learning how to set up a session including suggested safety procedures, tools and equipment, and horses. Many safety recommendations made in this chapter may be requirements by local Fire Marshals and/or Health Departments to meet code as a mental health and/or equine facility. It is strongly recommended to develop a good working relationship with local enforcement agencies and officials. They may be very influential in your EAP program's success.

Kersten (2000, September) suggests that the EAP treatment team go beyond the live demonstrations with family and friends. Invite the local law enforcement, fire department, rescue services, and medical clinics to the EAP program or practice, with one of the purposes being to advise and give consultation on safety concerns. They can help find and fix them, and help develop emergency plans for various crisis situations, such as fire evacuation, dealing with trespassers, or injury and medical attention. This is also a great opportunity to market the EAP program. You will be building relationships and selling your unique program to vital resources in the community. Not only will they learn about the fascinating and effective counseling services utilizing horses, but they will also have first-hand experience with the EAP team as quality, safe, and professional practitioners.

Kersten (2000, September) emphasizes that EAP professionals continue to be amazed at how effective these community resources can be to their organization. If a police officer, fireman, or nurse, etc. recommends your program, people listen! This also helps the team become more confident and secure in themselves, their community, and their profession.

Establishing a Safe Work Area

Fences, stables, paddocks, pastures, round pens, arenas, parking lots, and seating areas are all part of your work area and need to be maintained with safety in mind. All areas should regularly be checked for any signs of rot, decay, or damage. Holes, anywhere on your property, should be promptly and properly filled or blocked off from all access. Broken glass, wire, boards with nails, sharp objects or anything else that can result in a cut, puncture or scratch should be removed immediately and properly disposed of.

It is recommended that several fire extinguishers be kept available, up to date, and readily accessible in several very visible locations throughout your facility. The phone numbers of your local fire department, ambulance service, emergency vet service, and poison control center, along with the facility's barn address and directions on how to get there, should be posted in easy to read lettering at every phone as well as in a prominent place near your arenas and round pens. Because many therapy barns are located on back roads and rural areas, having the directions and address can mean the difference between life and death. Frequently, in crisis situations, basic information becomes difficult to remember. It is much easier and more accurate to read the information.

An up-to-date first aid kit for humans and another for horses should be available and easy to find, even for someone totally unfamiliar with your facility. It is strongly recommended in the field that there always be someone certified in first aid/CPR available. The American Red Cross provides first aid certification training and information. Safety training will help prevent the majority of accidents from even occurring, but EAP professionals need to be prepared just in case.

Safety around Arenas, Barns, and Corrals

Because stables and programs differ drastically in their horse areas, it is difficult to be specific about safety standards or expectations. This particular area requires observation, planning and common sense. In horse and therapy worlds, when it comes to safety you cannot leave any stone unturned. Kersten (April, 1999) recommends that the EAP team always be looking for unsafe or potentially dangerous areas of their facility or program. This means going through the facility with a fine-tooth comb.

Kersten (April, 1999) describes this EAP safety evaluation technique as the "t" in safety. This means that while the horse professional is going around the facility looking for safety concerns, he/she should use a vision pattern similar to that of the small letter "t". When beginning this walk around the barn, arenas, or corrals, start by looking up. Look up high for anything that may come in contact with the client's head or possibly the horse's head. Continue by making repairs or notes of what will be need to be fixed. As this search continues on, the horse professional should lower his/her head and look from side to side. Here he/she should be looking for objects sticking out that may come in contact with the client's or the horse's shoulders or sides. This includes nails, gate latches, etc. After the horse professional has made proper note of left and right, he/she will again drop his/her head and look to where the client's and the horse's feet will be traveling. Look for holes, rocks or uneven ground that may cause a person or a horse to trip or stumble.

These are the basics to the "t" in safety technique described by Kersten (April, 1999). It should be done routinely at the facility, and should be done at every entrance and exit to the EAP facility, arena, and pasture. Once the "t" has been completed from walking around on the ground, the horse professional should mount up on a horse and do the same wherever clients might ride, if there is a mounted component to the program. The same "t" observation aboard the horse will help the EAP team find those nasty little things that lead to both minor and major injuries to humans and horses.

Kersten (April, 1999) notes also that almost every facility, stable or ranch has some safety concerns that cannot be easily fixed or changed or make it 100% safe. For these things, it is recommended to mark the area with a bright color so at least a person is able to better see it. You may also use cones, tires, etc. to mark the area. Take time to do this both on the ground and on horseback. The EAP horse professional may be surprised at what he/she notices and has been luckily missed (Kersten, April 1999).

Again, I hope by now the treatment team is beginning to see a pattern here that each and every safety issue is an opportunity for growth for clients. Be creative with this. It can be a great activity to ask clients to investigate the barn for safety concerns and come up with solutions to fix the hazards using the same technique. This can also transfer into a good homework assignment to examine their home for safety and remedy the problems.

Tools and Equipment used in Facilitation

Many times, the treatment team brings their own equipment to a new facility but sometimes they may share equipment with others. The EAP team may even choose to simply use what can be found around the stables visited. Any of the discussed arrangements are acceptable, as long as, the EAP treatment team looks very closely at what is available because many items, however creative, can be used in a very unsafe manner (Kersten, 1999, July).

Boards/Logs/Poles

Boards, logs, and poles are very good items to be used for jumps, boundaries, make shift corrals, etc. It is important to inspect them for jagged edges or old, dry portions that can cause slivers in hands and horses. Store some well-treated painted poles at facilities you use or ask if you can paint and repair items at other facilities. Some EAP professionals prefer using PVC pipe rather than wood because it is light weight and doesn't splinter or need painting.

Old Used Tires

Because they are versatile, free, and smaller and lighter than other equipment, used tires are good to have. With tires, because they can be gotten free from a variety of tire stores, be selective. Check the condition of tires. Look for protruding steel wire in steel-belted tires. Also, check for screws, bolts, and other items sticking out. It is easy to cut a leg or hand with tires with these hazards, which really disrupts a session.

Figure 12.1 Props may be traditional horsemanship equipment but may also include non-conventional props. Props provide opportunities for metaphors so creativity is key.

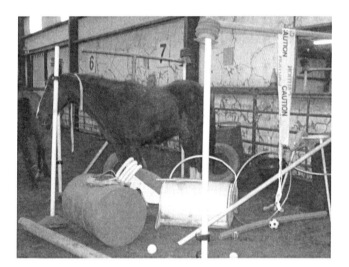

Ropes/Hoses/Cords

Many clients have never seen a rope, but in the passion of the creative moment, they will try and reenact their favorite western movie. Ropes, hoses, and/or extension cords get caught, tangled, and burn people and horses. Plus, the EAP treatment team runs the risk of someone or something getting dragged around.

It is argued within the field that all such items should be removed and not available for use. Other EAP professionals believe that these items are positive tools and when used properly are very helpful. These professionals state that any piece of equipment used inappropriately can become a weapon. This is the perfect opportunity to help the client learn respect for equipment and safety. Nevertheless, both professionals should consider the client's emotional and physical safety when determining whether or not a client is ready for such lessons to occur.

If these items are of concern, there are creative alternatives. Many EAP professionals have turned to ribbon, twine, or marking tape in place of traditional ropes. These options are chosen because they break if under strain; therefore, reducing the physical safety concerns that ropes can provide in some cases. These type alternatives create a different response with a horse than traditional ropes do. These alternatives provide unique metaphors and lessons about control, connection, and relationships.

Whips

Many training facilities have lunge whips or crops available for training horses. If people feel they need them for getting their horse's attention, that's a whole different issue. Kersten (1999, July) disputes the training tactic that whips are extensions of your arm. He, like many other EAP professionals, believes that in the hands of unfamiliar people, whips become tools of aggression. This perspective recommends putting them out of reach and out of sight.

The EAP treatment team must consider what the whip is a metaphor for and what the purpose of having the whip is for the activity and client. Especially when dealing with victims and victimizers, the emotional safety of a whip needs to be considered due to the metaphorical value it may hold for the client. Remember, EAP is not horsemanship.

Blindfolds

Blindfolds are very important to many facilitators in experiential activities. For therapeutic games and rope course activities, they assist in driving many points home.

Many EAP professionals use some form of blindfold during a horse activity. On some low level exercises, they may be marginally safer. Nevertheless, according to Kersten (1999, July), they increase potential injuries by 50% when used in Equine Assisted Psychotherapy. Take note of a blind folded person's mannerisms. They are quicker and more exaggerated in their movements which throw the horse's interpretation of safety off. The horse may act defensively, picking up on fear. In addition, the person cannot see the horse to push away or protect himself/herself from being bumped. EAP professionals opposing the use of blindfolds suggest that if they are needed, to do the blindfolded exercise prior to use of the horse. Also, it is suggested to remove other senses before limiting sight when possible. No matter what stance the team takes, the EAP professionals must consider the added risk of limiting sight for the client and consider that there may be other ways to achieve similar goals (Kersten, 1999, July).

Another use of blindfolds in Equine Assisted Psychotherapy is blindfolding the horse for leading and/or driving activities. However, this also increases the risk of injury, so it is important to know the horse's response to such an activity. It is recommended that the Equine Specialist try this with the horse prior to the client doing the activity.

Like any other prop or activity, the key to success is to be purposeful with the use of the blindfold and weigh the potential risk with potential benefits. Through appropriate horse choice and activity design, the risk can be decreased and lessons of trust, communication, faith, teamwork, and staying calm can be very powerful. The use of a blindfold in a haltered/leading activity would be very different than having a client blindfolded with horses moving freely around the arena. As a result, the team should continually be asking themselves if there is a safer way to explore the treatment goal; if so, choose that avenue.

Variety in Equipment and Therapy Horses

Creative and Therapeutic use of Props

As stated above, props and equipment vary as much as the EAP activities themselves. As stated by EAGALA (2012), EAP sessions are designed to be experiential, incorporate the horse as an active facilitator for change, and create a parallel to the clients' lives. Facilitators invite clients to participate in experiences which accomplish this design and address the clients' treatment plan, goals, and needs. The key view is to think of the session as providing an opportunity for the clients to tell their story. Activities provide the structure through which their story begins to emerge (EAGALA, 2012).

The space and props are all potential metaphors in the client's story so be deliberate in choosing them. It is useful to have various types of resources in the space to act as potential symbols for whatever may arise. EAGALA (2012) defines two types of symbols that can be represented in props:

> **"Abstract" symbols** are props that could mean anything for the clients, namely traditional props found in the arena. They can also be non-traditional props but have no direct meaning to the client going into the session
>
> **"Direct" symbols** are props that may relate directly to a client or group. For instance, for a group of corporate executives there might be a chair, desk, old computer, or phone.

Some of the traditional "abstract" symbols EAP professionals have often been known to use are items such as:

- Poles
- Cones/Tires
- Halters/Lead ropes
- Saddle/Blanket
- Lunge Lines/ Driving Lines
- Barrels & Jumps
- Brushes/hoof picks
- Hula hoops
- Sticky Pads/Markers/Finger Paints/Sidewalk Chalk
- Buckets
- Horse feed/hay
- Swim "noodles"
- Plastic colored balls
- Large beach balls
- Tarps
- Plastic bags/sacks
- Wheel Barrows
- Other traditional horse tack and gear

With metaphorical learning in mind, many professionals have chosen to add more non-traditional props to their arena as "direct" symbols. Items such as suitcases, backpacks, crutches, spoons, kitchen sink, mattress, toys, ribbon, exercise balls, weights, ball & chain. As portrayed in Figure 12.1, the options are only limited by the facilitators' creativity. The two most important determining factors when selecting props for each activity are: (1) the goals/objectives of the session and (2) safety. Some helpful questions to ask in this process may include: Do the props/equipment chosen create any safety concerns? If so, are these concerns such that they should be avoided or could some other prop provide the same metaphor with less risk?

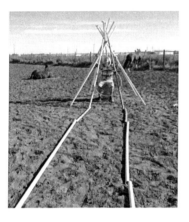

Figure 12.1 Allowing the client to create his/her story through the use of props can be very beneficial in progress. Leave creativity to the client.

Creativity in Therapy Horse Selection

EAP activities can be conducted with only one horse involved or a herd of horses – depending on client needs and activity design. A person interested in this form of therapy can begin work with only one horse. Nevertheless, having a variety of personalities and qualities to choose from within a herd adds much discussion, depth and variation to a session.

To work through treatment goals, it is at times beneficial to match a client to a horse with a similar personality. On the other hand, it is sometimes therapeutically beneficial to pair clients up with a horse that has a personality like someone they struggle to get along with. In addition, it also can provide valuable information to allow the clients to have a choice in which horses are chosen.

Therefore, the more horses available, the more options the treatment team has to choose from. Remember to keep in mind that every horse has the potential for being therapeutic. The question the horse professional needs to ask is: "Will the qualities of this horse contribute enough in EAP sessions to offset the cost of owning and/or maintaining the animal?" If not, the horse may not be the best fit for your program.

Horses vary in size, breed, and color. Many EAP professionals believe that there is not any living horse that cannot be used for EAP in some fashion. However, these professional agree that not every horse is appropriate for all activities and/or all clients. Other EAP professionals stand on the conservative end of this debate saying that the risk of jeopardizing emotional safety is not worth it. They promote using only very reliable and versatile horses. The example is posed, could a horse that has been severely abused exhibiting extremely aggressive behavior toward other horses and/or people be therapeutic for a client who has experienced similar abuse and behavior? Could an activity done with this abused horse be conducted giving an opportunity for the client to develop a treatment plan for the horse in how to help it heal from the hurts? This is a high risk horse; therefore, the EAP treatment team must weigh the risks with the benefits. The higher the risky behavior in the horse, the more critical it is to have a very skilled and competent horse professional involved in the treatment team. No matter which way the team falls on the continuum with this issue, it is critical that as a team they are in agreement as to what approach to take. A divided team is sure to generate countertransference and other pitfalls within a session.

Horse professionals need to consider the versatility in each EAP horse they own. Otherwise, the operating and feeding costs can easily become unmanageable to pay through EAP service fees. It is recommended to have at least one or two very reliable horses that can be used with any client. In general, the more expressive the horse, the more dynamic the metaphorical potential because awareness to body language is an important lesson the treatment team must work to stimulate in therapy.

In addition to horse variety for therapeutic value, having a herd of horses also allows the horse professional to give horses a break when they need one. This can be compared to any business. Oftentimes, a business can manage with only one employee. However, if that business gets too busy, the one employee will quickly become overworked and eventually burn out. Horses are no different. Allowing the horses a break from EAP from time to time is healthy and will pay off in the long run.

Guidelines in Setting up an Activity

Once the treatment plan is completed, the EAP treatment team begins determining what EAP activities will best meet the treatment needs. There are many really good EAP activities already in use by other EAP professionals which can be incorporated into your practice or the treatment team and/or clients can create their own. Oftentimes, an existing activity can be used with a little variation to better target the client's needs and/or the horses used.

It is very important to remember that no matter what EAP activity the treatment team designs, the client's main issues will arise. The only exception to this occurring is when the treatment team attempts to control the direction of the session rather than allowing the horse and client to take the activity where it needs to go.

When setting up an activity, the EAP treatment team needs to have a basic idea of the plan and layout of the activity and possible discussion. Nevertheless, the team must be flexible and willing to adapt to the process that takes place in the session. Most importantly, the team must remember that the purpose of the activity is to provide an opportunity for the clients to share more of their story. Both facilitators must let go of any expectations of outcomes and enter the arena with a curiosity about how this activity/opportunity will play out.

Once the activity has been created, often it is helpful to write this activity out and consider all factors involved. Smolowe, Murray, & Butler (1999) suggest the following subheadings to bring some structure to an activity description.

Type

This is an overall theme or target issue to add clarity and structure. The type is meant to reflect how the activity can be used but not limit the activity to only that use.

Group Size

Group size indicates the number of clients for which this activity is designed.

Horses

This section indicates the numbers or names of horses involved. This can be pre-selected by the treatment team or could be left up to the client as to who he/she wants to work with for the session.

Time Frame

This section indicates the length of time for the activity and debrief. Time frames can change based on the specific goal for the activity as well as other factors – group size, overall session length, etc.

Goals

This section indicates the treatment goals that the activity is providing opportunity to explore.

Materials

This section categorizes the props needed like a recipe. Be sure and consider the horses' reactions to such props. If a horse hasn't been exposed to a new prop, then it is recommended that the horse professional experiment with it to become more comfortable with their horses' responses (EAGALA, 2012).

Set-Up

Some activities require set-up before the session begins.

Briefing

This briefing period helps the group begin to see how the activity connects to the content of their therapy. It may be helpful to verbalize this portion, but often it is left for discussion afterwards.

Rules

This section gives step-by-step instructions for performing the activity.

Instructor's Notes

As an activity plays itself out, some predictable questions and pitfalls may occur. These notes offer tips for effectively facilitating the activity.

Variations

This section indicates some ideas for using an activity in a different way or for making the activity more or less challenging.

Debriefing

In this final stage of an activity, the facilitators conduct a dialogue around the activity and help the group to generalize and transfer their learnings while encouraging understanding of what happened, generalization and transfer.

Table 12.2 displays an activity designed (Mandrell & Mandrell, 2004) for a group of adolescents who are working on anger management. This layout gives the treatment team an idea of how an activity might look using Smolowe, Murray, and Butler's (1999) layout. This basic and straightforward format gives the EAP treatment team a thorough activity design with many flexible components.

This sample activity is intended to add detail to the understanding of an EAP activity design. Smolowe, Murray, & Butler (1999) state that thousands of activities and variations on activities can be used in an adventure design. The same can be said of EAP activities. In fact, the many adventure activities already designed can often be adapted to incorporate horses. The above activity is meant to offer but a brief glimpse into the possibilities within EAP. It needs to be incorporated as a live document always adjusting based on responses in the arena.

TABLE 12.2 HORSE SOCCER

Type: Anger Management

Group size: 2 – 8 clients

Horses: 2 horses -- One horse (to be the "soccer ball") & the other to allow opportunity for options/influence

Time frame: 30-45 minutes depending on group size

Materials: 4 cones or poles (to make goals), additional random props can be available in arena but don't need to be pointed out

Goals:
- Practice and examine anger management skills
- Explore impact anger has on success and relationships
- Examine problem-solving and creativity in presence of strong emotions

Setup:
Two groups placed on opposite ends of arena. Have two goals set up on either end of arena (poles or cones could be used as the goal) with additional props scattered around in arena.

Briefing:
This activity is to be a visual for how goals can be perceived to be very different and how that difference can sabotage success. Often it is beneficial to identify what the group's life goals are and label the "goals" as such.

Rules:
1. To get horse through their goal which is opposite them (like in soccer or hockey) as many times as possible in the amount of time designated
2. Basic 4 rules: can't touch the horse in any way, shape or form; can't coax it with food or pretend to have food; can't use a halter or lead rope; and can't leave the arena
3. Consequences of breaking rules are determined by the participants.

Instructor's Notes:
1. Did they assume they were competing and/or keeping score?
2. Were they sabotaging each other's success?
3. How creative are they? Did that change when they got frustrated?
4. What themes and patterns are present in their behavior? Any exceptions to behaviors or responses?
5. How did the horses respond?
6. Is there a way for them to have different goals and all be accomplished?
7. What causes frustrations and at what point does frustration turn into anger?
8. What do they do with their anger – is it motivating them to succeed or do they shut down?

Debriefing:
1. What was going on for them during that activity?
2. How did the horses respond to their approach?
3. What approach did they take to handling frustration in that activity?
4. What helped them to be successful or what held them back from feeling successful in the activity?
5. What life applications do they see in this experience?

© Refuge Services, Inc. Reprinted with permission

As discussed throughout this chapter, EAP professionals must use their tools to meet the specific treatment needs of their clients. In most cases, an adventure activity or activity type is customized to accomplish a specific set of outcomes (Smolowe, Murray, & Butler, 1999). With EAP, this is not always the case due to the fact that the horses have the ability to dramatically alter the outcome of the session. With this work, the purpose of the activity is to offer an opportunity to see the client(s) problem-solve, relate to others and self under stress, and experiment with new actions and solutions. If either of the facilitators enter into the activity with an outcome in mind or expecting to see it look a certain way, they will miss the opportunity to see the experience from the client's perspective and will struggle remaining fully present to the enlightening information being conveyed. As a result, each activity must be created with flexibility and as an exploratory tool.

Topics for Discussion:

1. *Design an activity and write it out using the suggested layout and subheadings explained in this chapter.*

2. *It was debated in this chapter as to whether all horses are suitable to use in EAP activities. Discuss your personal evaluation criteria on horse selection.*

3. *Once again safety is discussed. In this chapter, safety is talked about in the context of session preparation and setup. Discuss the safety considerations that need to be made regarding the activity you designed in question #1. Discuss your horse selection criteria as a part of this as well.*

4. *Evaluate the training facility you are using with the "t" in safety technique. Discuss your findings and possible remedies to any problems.*

CHAPTER 12

Chapter Notes

13 CRISIS RESPONSE

Objectives:
- **Identify crisis intervention and qualities of effective crisis intervention worker**
- **Describe a therapeutic crisis response**
- **Explore crisis prevention by reducing risk and liability**
- **Define reality safety**
- **Identify a recommended therapeutic crisis response**

In this chapter, Equine-Assisted Psychotherapy is compared to crisis counseling. Understanding the similarities helps you realize how important the EAP treatment team's response to each session is. We will explore characteristics of effective crisis intervention, as well as, qualities that describe a skilled EAP crisis response professional. We will also discuss a wide array of components that can minimize crisis situations and/or decrease damages as a result of an incident.

In essence, EAP structures activities that metaphorically represent difficult situations in a client's life. According to James & Gililland (2005), these challenges in a session are viewed as crisis moments. There are many definitions of crisis. To summarize these definitions, James and Gililland (2005) define **crisis** as a perception or experiencing of an event or situation as an intolerable difficulty that exceeds the person's current resources and coping mechanisms. Unless the person obtains relief, the crisis has the potential to cause severe affective, behavioral, and cognitive malfunctioning (James & Gililland, 2005). This is what EAP is all about. Therefore, this chapter will be focused on all the aspects of handling a crisis effectively – from reducing risk and liabilities to crisis intervention.

Crisis Intervention

Good crisis intervention, as well as good therapy of any other kind, is a serious professional activity that calls for creativity and the ability to adapt to changing conditions of the therapeutic moments. To that extent, crisis intervention at times is more art than science and is not always prescriptive (James & Gililland, 2005). Therefore, just as James

& Gililland (2005) caution, I will give the same warning -- there are no clear-cut prescriptions or simple cause-and-effect answers in this book as to how to handle crisis situations in EAP.

Crisis, left unattended to, can be a danger because it can overwhelm the individual to the extent that serious pathology, including homicide and/or suicide, may result. On the other hand, crisis that is attended to is an opportunity because the pain it induces compels the person to seek help (Aguilera & Messick, 1982). If the individual takes advantage of the opportunity, the intervention can help plant the seeds of self-growth and self-realization (Brammer, 1985). Discussing safety concerns as they arise with the client models addressing problems face on rather than avoiding the issue.

Clients can react in any one of three ways to crisis in an EAP session. Under ideal circumstances, many clients cope effectively with crisis by themselves and develop strength from the experience. They change and grow in a positive manner and come out of the crisis both stronger and more compassionate. Others appear to survive the crisis but attempt to block the hurtful affect from awareness, only to have it haunt them in innumerable ways throughout the rest of their lives. Yet others break down psychologically at the onset of the crisis and clearly demonstrate that they are incapable of going any further with their lives unless given immediate and intensive assistance (James & Gililland, 2005). In EAP sessions, professionals see first-hand the mini-crisis unfold and the client's choice of response in handling the crisis situation presented in the session. This gives the treatment team the opportunity to help redirect the client in discovering a healthier approach to resolving conflict. Successfully handing the crisis in session greatly increases the likelihood that the client will continue this new approach to crisis intervention in his/her personal life.

Life is a process of interrelated crises and challenges that clients confront or do not confront, deciding to live or not (Carkhuff & Berenson, 1977). In the realm of crisis, not to choose is a choice, and this choice usually turns out to be negative and destructive as demonstrated in EAP activities. Choosing to do something at least contains the seeds of growth and allows a person the chance to set goals and formulate a plan to begin to overcome the dilemma (James & Gililland, 2005).

Art of Crisis Intervention

Janosik (1984) explains how disequilibrium accompanies crisis, how anxiety is always present, and how this discomfort provides an impetus for change. Although uncomfortable, this discomfort is always present in crisis situations, even when a client is able to take the crisis situation positively and find strength. James & Gililland (2005) emphasize how a crisis worker and EAP professional must take intervention to the performing art level by guiding the client through this discomfort. A master of this art is going to have some combination of techniques, skills, and a good deal of the following characteristics.

Life Experiences. Life experiences serve as a resource for emotional maturity that, combined with training, enable professionals to be stable, consistent, and well integrated not only within the crisis situation but also in their daily lives. However, life experiences alone are not sufficient to qualify one to be an EAP professional and can be debilitating if they continue to influence the professional in negative ways. For instance, it is important not to confuse the experience of being injured in a horse-related accident with being an expert on horse-related accidents. Many people associate experience with expertise, and they are not the same. This holds true within the counseling realm as well (James & Gililland, 2005). For instance, a person who has been married several different times does not automatically become an expert in marriage (Kersten, 2004).

Poise. The nature of crisis intervention is that the professional is often confronted with shocking and threatening material from clients who are completely out of control. Creating a stable and rational atmosphere provides a model for the client that is conducive to restoring equilibrium to the situation.

Creativity and Flexibility. Creativity and flexibility are major assets to those confronted with perplexing and seemingly unsolvable problems (Aguilera & Messick, 1982). Although practice in tough role-play situations builds confidence, how creative EAP professionals are in difficult situations depends to a large measure on how well they have nurtured their own creativity over the course of their lives by taking risks and practicing divergent thinking (James & Gililland, 2005).

Energy and Resiliency. Functioning in the unknown areas that are characteristic of crisis intervention requires energy, organization, direction, and systematic action (Carkhuff & Berenson, 1977). Feeling good enough about oneself to tackle perplexing problems day after day calls for not only an initial desire to do the work but also the ability to take care of one's physical and psychological needs so that energy levels remain high. A crisis worker and EAP professional must also be resilient. By its very nature EAP has many "downs" where no matter how capable, no matter how committed, no matter what was tried or done, "success" was not achieved in the session. It is critical that the EAP professionals take care of themselves physically and psychologically and make wise use of their available energy (James & Gililland, 2005).

Quick Mental Reflexes. EAP crisis work differs from typical therapeutic intervention in that time is a critical factor. Time to reflect and mull over problems is rare in EAP sessions. The professional who cannot think fast and accurately is going to find the business very frustrating indeed.

Growth Potential. The EAP professional must have the potential and desire to grow and change. Remaining static is not an option. The crisis-helping relationship is reciprocal and is greater than the sum of its parts. The professional changes as a result of every contact with a client. Successful resolution of the crisis results in two products: (1) helping the client overcome the crisis and (2) effecting positive change in the professional as a result of the encounter.

Other Characteristics. Additional attributes include tenacity, the ability to delay gratification, courage, optimism, a reality orientation, calmness under duress, objectivity, a strong and positive self-concept, and abiding faith that humans are strong, resilient, and capable of overcoming seemingly insurmountable odds (James & Gililland, 2005).

Crisis Intervention Model

Even though human crises are never simple, James & Gililland (2005) have found that it is desirable for the crisis professional to have a relatively straightforward and efficient model of intervention. The six steps described below can be used as an action-oriented, situation-based method of crisis intervention in an EAP session. This six-step model presented by James & Gililland (2005) is the hub around which the crisis intervention strategies revolve in traditional counseling and EAP alike, and the steps are designed to operate as an integrated problem-solving process.

Assessing. The first three steps of (1) defining the problem, (2) ensuring client safety, and (3) providing support are more listening activities than they are actions. The final three steps of (4) examining alternatives, (5) making plans, and (6) obtaining commitment to positive action are largely action behaviors on the part of the professional, even though listening is always present along with assessment as an overarching theme.

Implementing. Steps 1, 2, 3 are essentially listening and observation. Steps 4, 5, 6 are all essentially involving acting strategies. Step 6 is obtaining a commitment – helping client commit to definite, positive action steps that the client can own and realistically accomplish or accept.

Planning. A plan should (1) identify additional persons, groups, and other referral resources that can be contacted for immediate support, and (2) provide coping mechanisms – something concrete and positive for the client to do now, definite action steps that the client can own and comprehend. The plan should focus on systematic problem solving for the client and be realistic in terms of client's coping ability. The critical element in developing a plan is that clients do not feel robbed of their power, independence, and self-respect. The central issues in planning are clients' control and autonomy. The reasons for clients to carry out plans are to restore their sense of control and to ensure that they do not become dependent on support persons such as the EAP professionals and/or horse.

Action Strategies for EAP Professionals

James & Gililland (2005) define a list of essential relationship skills that can be adapted to describe a skilled EAP professional, including attending, listening, communicating, showing empathy and acceptance, exhibiting genuine responses, and ensuring client safety. A number of action strategies and considerations may enhance the EAP professional's effectiveness in dealing with clients in crisis.

Recognize individual differences

The EAP team must view and respond to each client and each crisis situation as unique.

Assess yourself

At all times, EAP professionals must be fully and realistically aware of their own values, limitations, physical and emotional status, and personal readiness to deal objectively with the client and the crisis at hand.

Show regard for client's safety

The professional's style, choices, and strategies must reflect a continuous consideration of the client's physical and psychological safety as well as the safety of others involved. The safety consideration includes the safety of the EAP professionals, clients, and horses as well as the ethical, legal, and professional requirements mandated in counseling practice.

Provide client support

The EAP professionals should be available as support persons during the crisis period. They should work to help the client clearly define the problem through observations and questions. Many clients have multiple problems that can be very complex.

Consider Alternatives

In most problem situations, the alternatives are infinite, but crisis clients have a limited view of the many options available. Through the use of EAP activities and open-ended questions, elicit the maximum number of choices from the client.

Plan action steps

In crisis intervention, the EAP professional endeavors to assist the client to develop a short-term plan that will help the client get through the immediate crisis as well as make the transition to long-term coping.

Use the client's coping strengths

In crisis interventions and EAP in general, it is important not to overlook the client's own strengths and coping mechanisms. If they can be identified, explored, and reinstated, they may make an enormous contribution toward restoring the client's equilibrium and reassuring the client. The EAP team should attend to client's immediate needs. It is important for crisis clients to know that their immediate needs are understood and attended to by the EAP professionals. It is also helpful to use referral resources in crisis intervention and EAP.

Develop and use networks

Networking is having and using personal contacts within a variety of agencies that directly affect the ability to serve clients effectively and efficiently.

Get a commitment

A vital part of crisis intervention is getting a commitment from the clients to follow through on the action or actions explored in session to be practiced in their life outside the arena.

Legal Implications

In addition to the added risk of activities recreating crisis situations for the client, the use of horses adds another liability to this formula. All horses, no matter how kind, gentle and cooperative, do pose some risk to humans. The goal in any good risk and liability reduction program should be to limit those risks as much as is reasonably possible. To reduce risk and liability around the horses, one must also consider the mental and physical condition of the clients.

From a legal standpoint, keep in mind that no one can ever create a totally risk free environment. The treatment team's goal in regard to limiting risk and liability should be to:

- Follow the prevailing laws of the community,
- Have appropriate legal documents drawn up by qualified professionals
- Educate employees, partners, clients, families, volunteers and outside therapists of the law
- Stay alert for possible dangers
- Check and maintain equipment so that it is as safe and reliable as possible
- Learn and make sure employees, volunteers and partners learn first aid
- Establish a game plan for handling emergencies and make sure that your employees, partners, clients, families and outsider therapists are aware of these procedures.
- Make sure that everyone who works with the treatment team considers safety the number one priority.

Crisis Prevention

With regard to reducing risk and liability, EAP focuses primarily on one's mental state or emotional safety. In this chapter, we will term this philosophy "reality safety" as defined by Kersten (2004) because crisis intervention, within the realm of EAP, creates many fears of risks and liabilities within many EAP professionals.

By way of definition of terms, "**reality safety**" means real or true and actual, as opposed to ostensible, ideal, or imaginary. The path to becoming more "real" in our lives requires an ample amount of critical thinking, which is being more critical of what is being done and said by others, as well as ourselves. Being accurate in our perception and judgment of ourselves is the best place to start becoming healthier and safer with the horses in sessions, as well as, in life (Kersten, 2004).

Equine safety and training articles and books are written by people who are making an honest attempt to help. Nevertheless, people from this "reality safe" liability paradigm promote critical thinking when evaluating the benefits of such material. For instance, Kersten (2004) promotes further investigation into ideas and the questioning of oneself and others so that skills and beliefs are constantly being evaluated.

While all these preventative measures may not be able to prevent an accident from ever occurring on the property or with horse(s), they should reduce the likelihood of accidents and their severity. However, if an accident occurs, no matter what philosophy taken, impulse of human kindness, responsibility or regret may overcome the EAP professional, volunteers, employees or co-workers. Instead, an EAP professional skilled in crisis intervention might say, "What just happened there?" "Tell me about that?" "What life lessons are there for you in that experience?" or "Does that ever happen to you in life?" All of which are statements that express your empathy, observation, and presence. They focus on the emotional safety and therapeutic aspects of the incident, which are critical components in effective crisis intervention in an EAP session.

Prevention Planning

Kersten (2000, July/August) emphasizes that one of the fundamental components to EAP is safety – safety of the client, horses, and treatment team. EAP professionals don't rely simply on manufactured safety equipment to ensure safety in crisis intervention. Professionals should concern themselves with all the facets of safety including the physical and emotional safety of clients, partners, and horses. We cannot rely on a single piece of equipment to keep us all safe. Because of this, safety training and planning for each and every program or private practice is paramount not only for clients as discussed in the model of crisis intervention, but also from the perspective of crisis prevention for the EAP treatment team.

Along with the trainings and practice, planning is very important. Each and every program or practice should have an emergency plan. These plans should begin with the client in mind. The first day or session should involve filling out the necessary paperwork and agreements to allow the EAP professionals permission to get necessary care in the event a client is injured. Along with this, phone numbers and steps should be listed for others to assist if the situation presents itself. Reviewing these emergency procedures should be done frequently enough that it is second nature for everyone in the organization. It should be kept fresh in mind. With planning and practice, role model the following:

> Safety – for self, others, and concern for the future.
> Confidence – in self, the program, and practice.
> Ability – to influence the outcome of any situation.

Kersten (2000, July/August) reports that with confidence and the awareness the EAP treatment team gains through training and planning, they decrease chances of:

> Over-reacting to situations and making them even worse.
> Giving up attitudes in clients because of fear or a lack of knowledge of alternatives.
> Clients relinquishing responsibility to others to keep everyone safe

From a therapeutic standpoint, it is important and critical to remember that the treatment team's personal beliefs about safety and liability impact the way they conduct their sessions and respond to crisis. A treatment team should continually ask themselves before acting on a situation, "Is this intervention truly in the best interest of the client – both physically and mentally?" (Kersten, 2004).

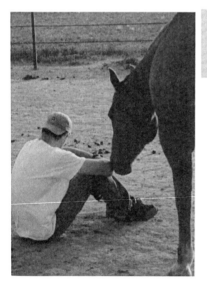

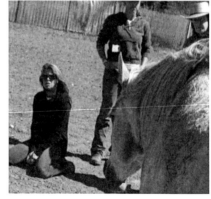

Figure 13.1
The horses are the most effective approach to crisis situations in most EAP sessions.

Topics for Discussion:

1. In this chapter, an EAP professional was compared to a crisis intervention counselor. Discuss this comparison.

2. Describe the techniques, qualities and skills explored in this chapter that define an EAP professional as someone who can become a master at crisis intervention?

3. List the essential relationship skills and action strategies necessary for an EAP professional to effectively handle any crisis situation?

4. In addition to being a skilled crisis intervention professional, what other considerations should an EAP treatment team consider in reducing risks and chances of a severe crisis situation occurring?

5. Describe a scenario where a crisis (physical, emotional, and/or both) has occurred during an EAP session. Explain the appropriate crisis intervention approach to working through this situation.

Chapter Notes

CHAPTER 13

Chapter Notes

14 COMPONENTS OF PROCESSING

Objective:
- **Identify four components of EAP processing**
- **Examine key questions to ask during therapy**
- **Assess the benefits of metaphors to retention**
- **Explore reasons to process**

Gass (1993c) defines **processing** as an activity that is structured to encourage individuals to plan, reflect, describe, analyze, and communicate about the activity. Processing can occur prior to, during, or after the experience. However, a wealth of valuable information is lost when you wait until everyone has completed a learning activity before asking clients to reflect and process (Luckner & Nadler, 1997). Adapted from Gass (1993a), who describes four general uses for processing an activity, processing EAP activities can be used to: (1) help clients focus or increase their awareness on issues prior to an EAP event or to the entire experience; (2) facilitate awareness or promote change while an EAP experience is occurring; (3) reflect, analyze, describe, or discuss an EAP experience after it is completed; and/or (4) reinforce perceptions of change and promote integration in clients' lives after the EAP experience is completed.

In this chapter, we will explore four components to consider when processing an EAP session. For maximum benefit, all aspects of the session must be considered. In EAP, the most common component overlooked is the horse. EAP professionals often find themselves focusing so much on the activity design and outcome or the person-to-person interaction and reaction that they miss the key insights their four-legged therapy partners have to offer. It will be important to remember that each component is equally important and works together to provide lasting change for clients. The processing of these components is critical in order to transfer changes made in session to conscious awareness necessary for this experience to be generalized.

Four Components of EAP Processing

Equine-Assisted Psychotherapy contains learning on many levels. There is so much going on in an EAP activity that it is vital for the treatment team to help sort out what is occurring during the processing time. Every EAP session contains four primary levels of abstraction that need attention. The first component is typically defined by the activity itself and the challenges it creates for the clients. Were they successful? How did they solve the problem? What resources did they use? While the second component is focused on the horse's response to the clients. How did the horses respond? What messages were the horses conveying to the clients through their behavior? Were the clients giving the horses mixed messages and, if so, how did the horses respond to that? The third component considers the clients' responses to the horses. Did the clients acknowledge that the horse had a role in the activity? Did they thank the horse for cooperating? Did they set limits and/or boundaries for the horse or did they just wait until the horse was ready? Finally, the last component takes into consideration the process that takes place within the group, family, and/or individual. How did the group plan? Were the opinions of each family member valued? Who made the final decisions? Which techniques were chosen, and why? How did they respond to one another and to the challenge itself? When clients became frustrated, what did they do? As explained in Figure 14.1, no component is necessarily higher or more significant than any other, they are simply all different perspectives necessary to consider.

One example that demonstrates these components is an EAP activity previously explained in Chapter 8 called "Life's Obstacles" (EAGALA, 2006). The goal of the activity is to get the horse over a small jump. The jump is placed in the middle of the arena. The group has 4 rules: They can't touch the horse, can't lead it, can't coax it with food or pretend to have food, and can't leave the arena. The most obvious means to achieve this goal are removed to create a challenging situation requiring problem-solving and communication. The lessons learned considering component one reinforce the ability to set a goal and achieve it, explaining the content of the session. Reviewing components two through four, the process of achieving the goal is considered. These levels reveal the fact that everyone has a part, the horse and each participant. All levels have value. All levels are part of the challenge and horse experience. The real goal is not only to successfully complete the challenge with the horse, but also to complete the challenge using skills and techniques that bring the group together and that reinforce the power of choice.

Figure 14.1 Components of EAP Processing

Component 1: The Activity
The first component is typically defined by the activity itself and the challenges it creates for the clients. Were they successful? How did they solve the problem? What resources did they use?

Component 2: What the Horse is Doing
The second component is focused on the horse's response to the clients. How did the horses respond? What messages were the horses conveying to the clients through their behavior? Were the clients giving the horses mixed messages and, if so, how did the horses respond to that?

Component 3: What the Client is Doing
The third component considers the clients' responses to the horses. Did the clients acknowledge that the horse had a role in the activity? Did they thank the horse for cooperating? Did they set limits and/or boundaries for the horse or did they just wait until the horse was ready?

Component 4: Interaction between Horse and Client
The fourth component takes into consideration the process that takes place within the group, family, and/or individual. How did the group plan? Were the opinions of each family member valued? Who made the final decisions? Which techniques were chosen, and why? How did they respond to one another and to the challenge itself? When the client became frustrated, what did s/he do?

Component One – The Activity

When considering the first component of evaluation, the EAP team must observe the content of the activity. This component emphasizes the actual actions that took place in the arena. This is probably the most obvious component to most EAP professionals. The team gives the client a task, and the EAP professionals are observing as to whether or not the client achieved that given task. Within this perspective, the EAP team is considering how the client attempted to complete the task given. A few questions to be considered when evaluating a session from this component might include:

> ➢ How did the client approach the problem presented?
> ➢ What resources did the client use to accomplish the task?
> ➢ Did the horse do what the client needed to be done?
> ➢ What steps did the client take to find success? If success was not found, what happened that kept the client from being successful?
> ➢ What did the client say during the activity?

Remember, component one is considering the content (actions and expressed thoughts) of the activity; while the components to come are looking more at the process (interactions and non-verbals) of how it was done. As a facilitator, this is all information. It is important to not get caught up in having any expectations of right vs. wrong or success vs. failure on how the task is to be completed. The facilitators are using the activity to gain observable information about the client based on what happens in the arena.

Component Two – What the Horse is Telling You

A couple of the most remarkable abilities of the horse are to recognize behavior patterns and to mirror human behavior. For the EAP team to be at peak effectiveness, they must make an effort to observe the horse's response to all activities and clients. Listed below are examples of questions the EAP team should be asking themselves and/or their client when evaluating a session to ensure that they do not miss the important lessons that are being revealed by the four-legged therapy partners:

> What non-verbal cues did the horse communicate during this activity?
> Are there any themes within the horse's response to the participants? Does the horse keep doing the same thing three or more times (patterns)?
> How did the horse(s) respond to any confusing and/or unclear expectations of the participants? What can that teach the participants?
> How were the horses treated by the participants before, during, and after the activity?
> How did the horses relate to one another? What lessons were in their interactions with one another that can relate to human interactions?
> What did you learn about each horse (personality, mood, etc.)? How can this insight help the participant deal with different people in their lives?

In order to gain the most accurate information from the horse member of the EAP team, it is vital that the horse professional is skilled and knowledgeable – not only about horses but about recognizing important horse cues. Additional tips to consider when evaluating an EAP session:

> Always be aware of even the most subtle body language messages. These messages are telling you something.
> Clients can't fool the horses. If they don't have clearly in mind what they want the horse to do, and what part of the horse they want to respond, the horse will mirror their confusion. The clients' body language tells ALL their secrets.
> A person who is afraid is not clear in his/her cues, so the horse gets confused.
> Horses are simple creatures with simple lives. Often people make life too complicated, which causes many problems. Learn from the horse, who is very good at taking care of its basic needs (Lyons, 1998).
> Everything a horse does is in an effort to meet a basic need. People are the same way. Although environmental factors have an influence on our decisions (as with horses), our behavior is not caused by them. All our internally motivated behavior is geared toward getting things we want that satisfy one or more of our basic human needs: belonging, power, freedom, fun, and survival (Corey, 1996).

There is a caution about verbalizing all that the horse is communicating. Some EAP horse professionals feel a need to accurately interpret for the client what the horse is saying with its body language.

CHAPTER 14

Remember, EAP is not horsemanship. Just as Greg Kersten stated so adequately in Kersten and Thomas (2004), "The difference between horsemanship and EAP is: horsemanship is be like me, EAP is be yourself" (p. 8). As a treatment team, be careful not to project personal feelings or beliefs onto the horse. Leave this up to the client for interpretation. This is where the facilitators begin learning about how the clients see their world. The client's interpretation provides an opportunity to view the world through the client's lens. For example, a horse is standing with his head low and ears forward, little movement. The participating group has him surrounded and working frantically to get him to move. They are being very loud with lots of movement. One member of the group comes over and says that they think the treatment team should make the group stop because the horse is getting upset and wants to be left alone. Is this an accurate reading of the cues the horse is giving? No, but that is not what is important in this moment because it is an accurate description of how that client was feeling at the time – his/her perception of the situation which is very revealing about how s/he responds to being crowded or pressured. This is an example of transference. **Transference** is the process whereby clients project onto the treatment team past feelings or attitudes they had toward significant people in their lives (Corey, Corey, and Callanan, 1998). Figure 14.1 is another example of transference in EAP as expressed through a client's poem about her EAP experience.

Transference is a significant aspect of EAP and can provide valuable information to the treatment team if approached properly. On the other hand, the team must be aware of their personal transference in order to keep the session from becoming about the treatment team and not the client. Therapist and horse people are both guilty of this. Be aware that it is normal to have responses to the clients and arena situations. Nevertheless, the caution is that a personal response may influence an EAP professional to misread horse behavior, to jump into the session sooner than necessary, or to end the session altogether prematurely. Just as Thomas (2012) emphasizes, all facilitators need to acknowledge and understand the issues that are surfacing in themselves. They can then be more conscious of how they respond and work with the client, and keep the focus on what the client needs. When the team is not aware of their own **countertransference**, the session will turn into therapy for themselves, and stop being about what the client needs. As defined by Corey, Corey, and Callanan (1998, 2011), countertransference is any projections by a member of the treatment team that can potentially get in the way of helping a client.

Component Three – What the Client is Telling You

During the activity, the therapist's main job is to watch the clients and how they handle the issue or task presented. The therapist must remember to look beyond the content and words. This is the power of experiential learning. The actions and problem-solving skills displayed by the participant are the best tools for self-discovery and change. Hargrave (1994) shares that "7% of communication is word-based, while 55% is body language-based and 38% inflection-based. This places 93% of communication on non-verbal. The key to authentic communication and discovery is not to be found in the words the clients use, but in their body language and inflection. EAP shifts the focus away from words and puts it on the area

Figure 14.2 Examples of Transference arising from an EAP session written in a poem form.

MY WILD HORSE MIND

Valentine, Katie, Stormy
Wild Horses
Running Freely
No Boundaries
"Free" or is it Bondage?

My Thoughts
Wild Mind
Running Freely
Spinning, Spinning, Spinning
No Boundaries
"Free" or is it Bondage?

Wild Horses
Running freely throughout foreign neighborhoods
No container, no safety
Scared, Frightened, Paranoid, Confusion
Is this Really Freedom?

Wild Mind
Bolting at every second
Spinning out of control
Making up storyline after storyline
Chaotic
Scared, Frightened, Paranoid, Confusion
Is this really Freedom?

The Horses are caught
They are compassionately subdued and tamed
Led back to their safe "container"
They relax into calmness
They are now truly free
To be in their natural state
To be who they really are.

My Mind is caught by the Awareness
Of the present Moment.
My thoughts are compassionately subdued and tamed
My Mind is led back to a safe container
Called the Present
This very precious moment; like no other moment
My mind is Free to relax into its natural state
A state of openness, clarity, and strength
I am now Free to be who I really am.

Author remains anonymous to protect privacy

where accurate communication exists – body language of the horse and client. The EAP activities give the treatment team a more honest picture of the client's true messages and issues, while providing the client an opportunity to challenge life-coping skills.

Some important questions for the therapist to consider regarding the client's non-verbal communication and behavior in the EAP session are as follows:

> - What non-verbal messages did the client communicate during this activity?
> - Were there any themes or patterns within the client's responses to the activity and/or horses? Did the client do anything more than 3 times during the session?
> - Were there any exceptions to the client's behavior patterns?
> - What mixed messages did the client give during the activity? How did these affect the activity?
> - Did the body language of the client match the words verbalized by the client?
> - What role did the client play?
> - How did the client handle success? Failure? Disappointment? Discouragement? Etc.
> - How creative was the client in completing tasks and addressing problems encountered?

These questions are just a few examples of the many questions that should be considered when evaluating the process relating directly to clients' responses.

Component Four – What is the Interaction between the Horse and Client Revealing

In addition to the messages of the horse and the client, the interaction between the two must be considered in the evaluation of an EAP session. These interactions can give the team valuable information about how the client handles relationships and/or how the client handles difficult situations in life. The evaluation of the interaction needs to be considered in the context of each session, its tasks, and the metaphors that evolve naturally or by intent during the session. For example, the horse represents a male client, and the task is to get the horse over the jump. How the client treats that horse may be a good indication as to how the client feels about himself and/or what methods this client would like others to take when approaching him. On the other hand, if the horse represents "fear," then the approach this client takes might give the treatment team valuable insight into how he approaches fear in life. These interactions and their meaning are critical to the process of reflecting this experience back to the client's life.

A few questions to consider when evaluating a session based on the interaction between client(s) and horse(s) are as follows:

> - What patterns within the interaction between horse and client were there during the activity?
> - How did the client relate to all interactions in the arena?
> - How did the client treat the horses and/or other participants before, during, and after the activity? When things went well? When things didn't go well?
> - What means did the client use to communicate needs and wants while interacting with others and/or the horses? How was this received by all involved?
> - What themes were present in how the client approached the horses or others in the activity?
> - What life metaphors were represented in the interactions in the arena?

Prioritizing and Filtering Observations

SPUD'S is a framework developed by EAGALA (2006) to assist facilitators in where to focus observations since there are so many components to observations. While observing, there is a vital need to be free from the facilitators' agendas, judgments, biases, and beliefs; so the clients can express their perspectives and discover their own solutions (Thomas & DiGiacomo, 2013). Thomas and DiGiacomo (2013) explain the EAGALA trademarked SPUD's acronym as follows in Figure 14.3.

Figure 14.3. EAGALA's SPUD's ™

S – Shifts: Watch for any shifts that occur in behaviors, including actual physical placement, of both horses and humans. For instance, the horses were standing, now they are running (i.e. no movement in the horses to quick movement, horses standing near client to horses standing far away from client. Clients tend to do same thing.)

P – Patterns: If a behavior occurs three or more times, it is considered a pattern. These patterns tend to parallel other patterns in the clients' lives. (i.e. horses circling, horse comes to same spot over and over, horses are walking in straight lines. Client approaches horses from the right every time)

U – Unique: When observing, if the horse does something out of the ordinary, like kick up, or something dramatic or unusual, or if the humans do something that is unique to their behavior, note that moment. Note the unique behavior and what was happening in the entire arena with horses and humans in that moment. (i.e. horse walks up to client and puts nose under arm—this horse typically is very distant from people)

D – Discrepancy: This is referring to moments when verbal communication of the client does not match non-verbal actions of the client. For instance, the client says she "doesn't want to do this," but at the same time, she is walking towards the horses. The treatment team's primary reason for paying attention to these discrepancies is not to identify distrust in the clients. Observing these moments is important because it indicates an opportunity for change and a potential metaphor. (i.e. client says they are terrified of horses yet walks up to the horse with smooth and steady pace and strokes the horse...petting it all over body with fluid movements)

'S – Self-awareness or "My Stuff": While observing the experience of the clients and horses, the treatment team constantly observes their own countertransference. (i.e. facilitator notices that the client begins to remind him/her of a beloved cousin who had passed away recently from cancer. This client is coming because of similar circumstances)

EAGALA (2006) developed and trademarked a framework to assist facilitators in organizing observations in EAP sessions. This term is an acronym known as "**SPUD'S**." The 'S stands for "our stuff" (also known as countertransference) and our self-awareness of it. Thomas (2011) believes that the treatment team needs to observe themselves while observing all that is happening with clients and horses. She states that our beliefs, personality, past experiences and mood will influence what the treatment team focuses on and how the team chooses to intervene in a session (Thomas, 2011).

Value of Metaphors

A **metaphor** can be understood as one thing conceived as representing another. A metaphor includes symbols, different objects or elements that make up the metaphor creating a word picture (EAGALA, 2012). Word pictures can give powerful and poignant expression to the transfer of equine-assisted psychotherapy experiences back to life. Research has consistently shown that word pictures tap into the memory on a deeper level than auditory learning does. As mentioned before, it has been estimated that we remember only 20% of what we hear and 50% of what we see. We retain fully 80% of what we do (Smolowe et. al., 1999). As a result, there is great momentum for understanding the nature and power of EAP, and how it can make use of the way the human nervous system is wired to learn.

EAP gives the client a visible metaphor that can be applied to life experiences and relationships. Using these metaphors in session can enhance the lasting therapeutic effect for a client. Experiences in the arena may metaphorically represent a client's life in some way. Metaphors allow the client to connect the learning done in the arena to other areas of life outside the arena (EAGALA, 2012). Clients frequently see for themselves the metaphorical links between elements of the experience and issues that they are working on in themselves (Peel & Richards, 2005). These metaphors teach relational and coping skills as well as alternative ways to respond to difficult situations in life. For example, after struggling with the halter, a client finally gets it on and now is processing the experience with the treatment team. The client is wrapping the lead rope around her hand quickly and nervously. What might this mean for this client? What might the lead rope be in her life? Possibly, something she gets all wrapped up in or makes her feel all tied up in knots? Let the client decide the answer. Nevertheless, the metaphor connects the visual image of the lead rope wrapping around her hand to words, which has a more lasting impact on the human brain than traditional talk therapy does.

Everything in a session is a potential metaphor – people, horses, equipment, physical placement, patterns, feelings, treatment team, etc. Once the metaphor is established, continue to use it. It is not an arena or horse; it is now the environment and whatever the horse represents in the client's stated metaphor. Begin to look at everything from this perspective. An example is a horse that is identified by the client as a particular person and continues to be 'named' as that person through the sessions to follow (EAGALA, 2012).

Without this generalizability to life situations, a specific experience in EAP is merely an interaction with a horse. So, it is critical for the team to process the metaphorical value in an activity with a client and apply to the issues or problems the client is attempting to address. Some important aspects to ask yourself when processing or considering what metaphors are being presented:

> ➢ Ask the client what metaphors and/or applications to life they find in doing this activity?
> ➢ What can the horses represent in the activity? The activity goal? The obstacles? The props and/or tools that helped the client to accomplish the goal?
> ➢ With the lessons learned in this activity, now what? What did the activity teach you about life? What worked and what didn't work in the activity? How is that significant in real life?
> ➢ What parallels does the activity hold? How did the client handle frustration? Help? Boundaries? Obstacles? How does that relate to real life?

The questions can go on and on, but the most important question is the first one. It is critical to allow clients to tell their story and/or create their own meaningful metaphors before the team lays their observations and assumptions out for them. The clients must have the freedom to get out of the activity what they need. This will help further retention and impact when the clients are able to find the answers. Be cautious once again that the teams' personal agenda and counterference doesn't get in the way of clients getting what is needed from the activity.

Two types of metaphors

As described by EAGALA (2012), there are two types of therapeutic metaphor models that can be utilized in treatment: non-directive (natural and client-led) and directive (formal and goal-led). Both play an important role in treatment:

> **Non-directive** – when the facilitators recognize a metaphor being created naturally by the client (s) or ask the client to develop a metaphor based on the experiences of the client with the horses in the present moment.
>
> **Directive** – when facilitators set up the metaphor deliberately to match treatment goals with the horses as central to the metaphor construct. This is effective especially with single session clients or growth and learning clients, such as corporate groups.

An example of a non-directive metaphor would be a metaphor that surfaces in the moment. For instance, let's say the equine specialist observes the horse moving away from the client each time client reaches out her hand and asks the client about that. Client responds, "The horse doesn't want me to be close to him, just like my dad." This horse now represents her dad. The treatment team now takes the lead of the client with this non-directive metaphor and asks any further questions about horse behavior using "Dad" as a reference rather than "the horse" label. On the other hand, an example of a direct metaphor with this same client could be as follows: Today we want you to work with the horse that you said was like your "Dad" and build something in the arena to represent what you want your relationship to look like and take "Dad" there. In this instance, the direct metaphor is set up at the onset based on treatment goal to improve relationship with Dad. However, how this metaphorical opportunity plays out is left to the client's experience. Questions around observation of the activity in this case would reflect the direct metaphor rather than using terms such as "obstacle" or "what she built." It is "what she wants her relationship to look like." The treatment team could go even further and have the client describe what all the components of this desired relationship that she built represent.

Thomas and DiGiacomo (2013) believe that one of the most important qualities of a facilitator is the ability to be sincerely and genuinely curious. By being truly curious, the treatment team is able to learn and accept others rather than place judgments and expectations on them. The key as a facilitator is to be curious and never make any assumptions about the verbal or nonverbal messages of both clients and horses. All the observations and metaphors are intended to be used as opportunities for the clients to tell their story in more detail. This will help the facilitators in supporting a key foundation to EAP, the client's story. It is through this story that clients gain insights into current beliefs and behaviors, and direct where their stories (lives) go next (Thomas & DiGiacomo, 2013). All components of the experience in the arena have the possibility to serve as characters/symbols in the client's story – horses, props, the space itself, and anything that comes into the space. The facilitators need to allow the opportunity for the clients to engage in their stories and allow it to be the clients' story rather that "the facilitator's story." For example, Figure 14.4 tells a story. Depending on who's story is being told, the outcome and life application will be different.

Why Process?

Disequilibrium is a major catalyst for change. This is true not only for individuals, but for families and other groups as well (Luckner and Nadler, 1997). Luckner and Nadler (1997) continue to explain that "it is in this brief moment(s) prior to a unique action or 'breakthrough' that the ingredients for change are found. Here in these moments also resides information that will facilitate the transfer of learning from this success to other successes" (p. 28).

Figure 14.4 Who's catching who in this activity?

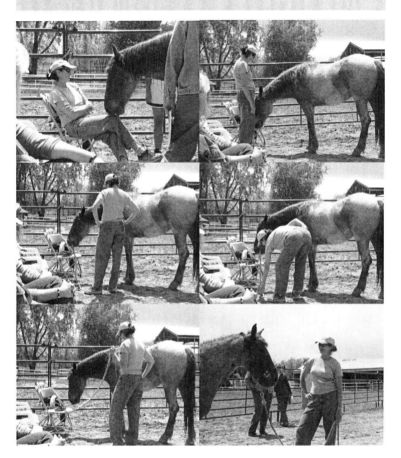

One aspect of EAP is asking clients to do something that they have never done before, entering into unknown territory away from their safety zone. In actuality, it's the struggle of the journey between the known and unknown where the "pearls" for future learning reside (Luckner & Nadler, 1997). It is at the edge of the breakthrough where processing the experience is most important as depicted in Table 14.1. As clients get closer to this unknown, new territory, their sense of disequilibrium increases and a sense of uncertainty exists. The wall of defenses and habitual patterns become prominent in an effort to control the sense of disequilibrium. Clients' feelings intensify at the edge; they may be fearful, anxious, confused, excited, or feeling alone (Luckner & Nadler, 1997).

Table 14.1-- Levels of Processing Diagram

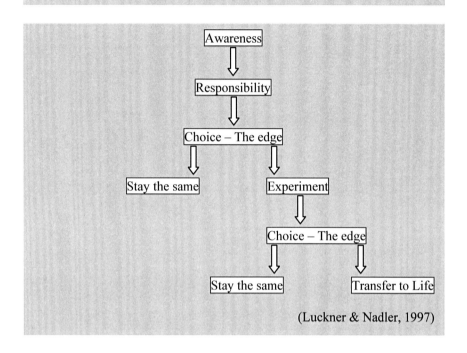

(Luckner & Nadler, 1997)

Learning takes place in an EAP session before doing the activity, during the activity, and after completing the activity. It is common to process the activity at the end of the session or upon success. This is very valuable yet can be greatly enhanced when we explore what happened right at the moment(s) before the success. Usually these moments pass quickly without the awareness of clients and are generally lost for current and future learning (Luckner & Nadler, 1997). Luckner and Nadler (1997) advocate putting these moments at the edge under a microscope and examining the feelings, patterns, conversations, physiology, beliefs, support, and metaphors that encompass these moments. The treatment team wants to slow down or freeze the moments before the success or the retreat, so that clients' thoughts, feelings, and actions that make up their strengths and/or weaknesses become conscious and both internally and externally communicated.

When this is accomplished, golden nuggets are valuable as new edges in other settings are approached (Luckner & Nadler, 1997).

The treatment team can never predict what will take place in the arena if they are trusting the process by staying present and observing. In each case, the horses show specific behaviors often not seen before, and may never do it again. They do what is important for each participant at that particular time in that client's treatment. If careful and consistent observation of the horses is not primary focus and instead the team focuses only on accomplishing the activity the way the team thought it should be done, the opportunity to experience a moment of new awareness and healing for the participant may be missed. As Connett (2008) concludes, if the team does not give the equine partners equal opportunity to direct the session when they so spontaneously sense the need, the most potent therapeutic moments may be missed.

Topics for Discussion:

1. *The client interprets the horse behavior as one thing and you disagree because you are familiar with horse cues. What do you do? Explain your response.*

2. *Discuss how to handle the client that doesn't see that anything he/she is doing with the horse relates to life.*

3. *Take the example given in the chapter – a horse is standing with his head low and ears forward, little movement. The participating group has him surrounded and working frantically to get him to move. They are being very loud with lots of movement. One member of the group comes over and says to you that they think we should make the group stop because the horse is getting upset and wants to be left alone. Is this an accurate reading of the cues the horse is giving? How should the team respond? What valuable information did you learn about the group? Discuss the answers to the proposed questions.*

4. *In this chapter, transference and countertransference are discussed. What are countertransference and transference?*

What role does awareness play in both? Which should the treatment team work to avoid? What might they look like in an EAP session? Give more examples.

Chapter Notes

Chapter Notes

15 PLANNING SESSIONS

Objectives:
- **Identifying the functions of a treatment plan**
- **Considering client goals when planning a session**
- **Exploring activity design**
- **Discussing impact of horse selection on session success**

After learning about all the key factors that come into play simultaneously in an EAP session, it is time to start putting all this information together. This chapter will discuss the topics to consider as a treatment team after the assessment of client issues has been completed. It is important, at this stage, to discuss as a team the plan of action in how to address the issues that have been identified. This chapter will explore a treatment plan format that can be adapted to EAP and other components that must be considered when setting up future sessions to address the clients' needs. These therapy goals should be determined jointly by the client and counselor, bringing together the client's unique perspective and the counselor's expertise and objectivity (Young, 1992). Being that EAP is a solution-focused approach to therapy, it is important to have an idea of where the client wants to be upon termination of therapy.

Incorporating Client Goals into the Session

Client goals should be considered when planning each session. This step will vary depending on the type of session (EAP vs. EAL), whether individual, family, or group. Often with groups, the goals are more generalized; nevertheless, the group's goals are to be considered when creating an equine-assisted activity.

One of the first steps in treatment planning is gathering information from the client as to his/her goals for treatment. With this initial information as a foundation for future planning, the treatment team (therapist and horse professional) is able to begin brainstorming activity options to address these issues.

Once this initial plan has been developed, the treatment team is able to present activities specially designed to help address the issues at hand. A caution in all planning is to not become too rigid with the order of activities or the goals for the session. The therapist and horse professional need to remain open to allowing the client to discuss whatever issues may be urgent in his/her mind that day, even if it seems to be different from the initial plan. Also, be aware that the presented issues to be addressed may often be mere symptoms of an underlying issue. The client's goals may change as the client becomes more aware of thoughts, beliefs, and behaviors.

After having done this type of therapy for several years, I am reminded over and over that the issues that need to be addressed will always arise in an activity despite the activity design. As a result, a tip to all treatment teams to remember when conducting sessions and planning activities – the main issues will come forth no matter what activity is presented to the client. So, with that knowledge, the treatment team need not get discouraged if an activity does not turn out as desired or if the activity must be changed at the last minute because a client has a new issue to discuss or work through. If the initial issue was a big deal, it will come up anyway. If not, it can wait – the therapist needs to address the issues that reveal themselves first because they are the biggest obstacles for the client at this point. It is important to allow the client and horses to lead the activity rather than the formation being rigid in how an activity needs to look

Young (1992) states that activities are a visual way of changing problem statements into workable goals and accomplishments. This statement describes precisely the purpose of EAP activities. Egan (1990) describes this process as helping the client move through four stages:

> - Declaration of intent
> - Mission statements
> - Specific aims
> - Concrete and specific goals

Stage 1: Declarations of Intent

At this stage, the client shows an interest in changing something in his/her life. In the early stages of EAP, the treatment team is exploring, observing, assessing, and establishing the supportive relationship which provides valuable information as to the client's desire to change. Quickly in EAP activities, the treatment team and client shift gears and begin the work of implementing change.

Stage 2: Mission Statements

Now that the problem has been isolated, the next step is to change the problem into a goal statement. The treatment team helps clients develop mission statements by pointing out observations with the horses and discussing how they handled situations in the arena. Then the team help the clients put that back into life.

Stage 3: Specific Aims

Now that the client has experienced some positive outcomes, the third step in boiling down the problem is what Egan (1990) calls "specific aims". The treatment team can facilitate movement from mission statement to specific aims quickly by restating the client's goals more specifically based on experience with the horses and asking the client to about this relation. Second, the treatment team asks the clients to explore in more depth the important aspects of their issues based on the activity.

Stage 4: Concrete and Specific Goals

The fourth stage Egan (1990) identifies is concrete and specific goals. In this final stage of the boiling down process, the treatment team asks the client to identify, in more detail, the conditions under which therapy would be considered complete. An important aspect to this is helping the client determine whether or not his/her goals are realistic.

All four stages occur very quickly in an EAP format compared to traditional therapy where this process may take several sessions. One of the advantages to EAP is that looking at the problem is a very brief portion of the process and the shift quickly turns to focusing on the solution and problem solving once the goals are identified. All of which may occur within the first assessment session.

Goal setting is seen as a critical step in cementing the therapeutic partnership and in transforming the focus of counseling from problems to solutions (Young, 1992). This occurs very naturally in an EAP session. Through the process of establishing mutually acceptable goals, the treatment team involve the clients in the process of finding their own solutions. Finally, the setting of goals helps both clients and treatment team anticipate the conclusion of therapy as a time when goals have been reached. Clearly, there are several skills that the treatment team must consider in order to help clients transfer the workable goal statements, or solution-focused skills, back into their life. The horses aid in boiling down client statements into specific aims.

Treatment Planning

Treatment planning involves selecting specific techniques or strategies to accomplish client goals. Treatment strategies are the steps to be taken in reaching these goals. Many agencies may have a treatment plan format that they recommend for their team; nevertheless, whether EAP or traditional therapy, the same format can be used. EAP is a legitimate therapeutic intervention and should be treated with the same degree of professionalism. Nevertheless, this may be new territory for the horse professional to be involved in. It will be important for the therapist to help coach the horse professional through this process. This treatment plan is a team effort; the horse professional's insight into the horse's behaviors and cues is vital to the design of treatment plan interventions.

One format the treatment team might use is the diagnostic treatment planning model known as DO A CLIENT MAP assessment (Seligman, 1990). Seligman (1990) describes her model as being similar to an hour-glass: a wide variety of assessments are made that then narrow to a single diagnosis that, in turn, broadens again into a number of intervention strategies. The diagnostic treatment planning model is an acronym: DO A CLIENT MAP. Filling out each portion of the client map is the method for completing a treatment plan. Table 15.1 below shows the elements of the plan adapted from Seligman (1990).

Designing Activities Related to Goals

Table 15.1 Outline of DO A CLIENT MAP

Elements of the Model	Description
D – Diagnosis	DSM – V diagnosis of all axes and/or presenting issues
O – Objectives	Goals of treatment
A – Assessments	Assessments needed (e.g. testing)
C – Clinician	Treatment team characteristics that would be helpful in treatment
L – Location of treatment	For example, inpatient versus outpatient
I – Interventions	Specific treatment strategies and EAP activities based on issues presented and diagnosis
E – Emphasis of treatment	For example, EAP versus traditional talk therapy (can specify theoretic approach)
N – Nature of treatment	Individual, couple, group, family
T – Timing	Frequency, duration, and pacing of therapy sessions
M – Medications needed	Need for medication evaluation by medical personnel
A – Adjunct services	Referrals, support groups, education
P – Prognosis	Amount of change or improvement expected with the presented issues

    Designing activities for clients is often a challenging step for beginning facilitators. This seems to be so difficult because for starters, the designer is often trying so hard to simulate the scenario in so much detail that it becomes too complicated. Keep the activity very simple and open ended and then build from there. Some good questions to consider when designing an activity are as follows:

TABLE 15.2   Activity Design Questions

> ➤ What are the goals of the client for this session? Remember to narrow it down to one or two issues at a time. It can get too overwhelming for the client and treatment team if you try to address too much too fast.
> ➤ What might aid in client's exploration of therapeutic issues to encourage insight, change, or closure? For example, a sexual abuse victim wants to work on trust issues and building healthy relationships. Allowing the client space to explore what building trust might look like for her. She might also benefit from exploring body language as it relates to honest communication.
> ➤ What experiences with the horses might help the client discover the new insights needed?
> ➤ Think about a game or activity you have experienced in education or play? Is there any way you can adapt that activity to incorporate horses to address these issues? For example, horse soccer came from the concept of soccer but using the horse as the ball with different instructions or rules.
> ➤ Many times it may be more therapeutic for the client to create his/her own activity or tell his/her story using the horses.
> ➤ Remember, the main issues are going to arise in whatever activity you choose, so don't get too bogged down in this process. The treatment team can build off of whatever is started in the activity. The power of this type of therapy is allowing the process to be in control, not the treatment team.
> ➤ Trust your horses to bring out the issues necessary. The team's job is to observe and reflect back to the client what happened and discuss change that took place and/or help the client discover what changes may need to take place. Overall, the team is to provide a safe place for the client to experiment with the changes in sessions to come.

Choosing the Appropriate Horse and Setting

As the treatment team is deciding on the activity based on client's presenting issues, the horse professional can contribute by helping interject the appropriate horse(s) to the activity. The horse professional needs to consider client goals and consider which horse(s) may provide best opportunity to explore these goals. Be mindful of what each horse might represent in the activity. If a horse has already been identified as a representation to something/someone in the client's life, the opportunity to further explore that relationship needs to take precedence over a new activity requiring a new horse(s) or setup.

In addition to the horse, the horse professional needs to consider the appropriate setting and setup for an activity. Always keeping safety in forefront of mind, the horse professional's job is to aid in determining the best setup for the activity presented. The number of horses used will influence the size of the pen needed for the activity. From past experience, a rule of thumb that has served well for us in keeping the clients safe is not using over five horses in an arena at a time (especially with groups), unless there is more than one horse professional. Too many horses can be overwhelming for the horse professional and heighten safety concerns for the clients in the arena. There can be too much activity to observe for one horse professional and therapist. Now, if the horses are in a large pasture and spread out considerably, this is not as big of an issue. Just remember safety – it is very important to give the horses enough room to interact without running over someone. Also, the horse professional needs to consider the clients and their level of comfort and experience with the horses. If it is a first session verses their eighth session, the horse chosen may vary. The client may be ready for a bigger challenge and able to read the horse's body language better.

Filtering out Personal Agendas

EAGALA (2012) states that projections based on our experiences occur all the time in everyone's lives. If people don't have knowledge from the past to project on what is around them, they wouldn't get very far! For that fact, it is also occurring in EAP sessions with clients and can be useful. However, the treatment team needs to be aware of how to use it. Therapeutic concerns occur when the EAP team's own projections, whether they are on clients (known as counter-transference), horses, or co-facilitators, remain in the pre-awareness stage. Pre-awareness projections have the potential to interfere with effective sessions. The less negative impact occurs for the client when the treatment team is more aware of personal projections. During EAP, the same process that is transforming for the client as they are working through situations to create better awareness in order to lead to change needs to be occurring personally within each treatment team member as well. New awarenesses within the treatment team lead to improved interventions and facilitating. The caution is that this process must not become focus of the session. After session debriefings or supervision can be very helpful for the treatment team to verbally sort out new awarenesses. EAGALA (2012) charts this filtering process with the following self-awareness diagram depicted in Table 15:3.

TABLE 15.3   Filtering Self-Awareness Diagram

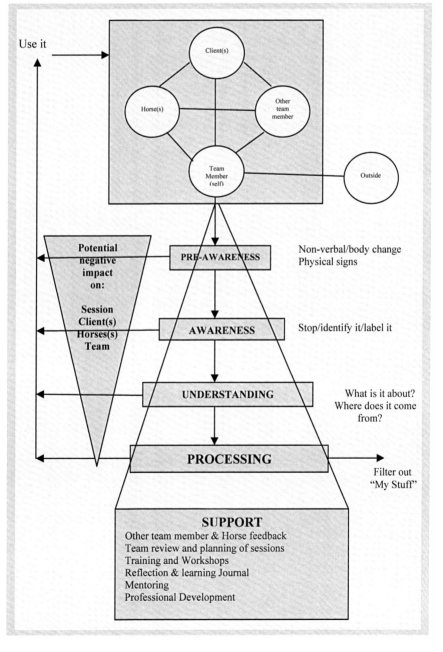

CHAPTER 15

At this point, the treatment team is ready to begin putting all components together to develop a treatment plan for the client. Remember, treatment planning is the art of selecting treatment strategies and activities once therapy goals have been identified and negotiated (Young, 1992). The horses are vital to the treatment plan's success. However, in order to access this information and insight, the treatment team must be skilled in allowing the process to happen rather than working to personally control the direction of the session. Use what occurs to be therapeutically beneficial and the team will have a healthier and more confident client in the end. Remember, the team's goal is to help the client deal with an ever-changing and unpredictable world with confidence and competence. There is no better practice than allowing the client to experience that truth in the safe surroundings of the arena.

Topics for Discussion:

1. Practice writing an EAP treatment plan using the DO A CLIENT MAP technique on the following possible client diagnosis:
   - Attention Deficit Hyperactivity Disorder (ADHD)
   - Major Depression
   - Eating Disorder – Anorexia
   - Drug/Alcohol Addiction

2. Design an activity that could be incorporated into one of the above treatment plans. You should include a name, setup, objectives/goals, instructions, rules, points to observe, and possible questions.

3. Compare the treatment planning process of EAP to traditional therapy. What aspects are similar? What makes them different?

Chapter Notes

16 FACILITATING SESSIONS

Objectives:
- **Examine the impact session design has on outcome**
- **Discuss the process of turning goal setting into goal implementation**
- **Explore session set up, activity design, and follow-up**
- **Illustrate examples of case note format**
- **Consider how much time is needed for client sessions**

As we continue to piece together the components that work in unison to orchestrate an EAP session, the visual image of how a session works should be coming into view for the reader. In this chapter, a discussion will include details about what is next once the treatment goals have been established with the client. This chapter will take the treatment team through the working stage of the EAP experience toward termination. During this time frame, the EAP team is actively designing and organizing activities to meet the treatment goals while keeping track of the progress made.

The EAP experiences are the critical link between the vision and realization of a client's goals. The activities lay out the contours of the client's potential new structure, which may be a groundbreaking creation or an addition to an existing structure. Either way, the activities must address, accommodate, and juggle multiple considerations. Most importantly an EAP activity design, like other adventure designs, must rest upon a firm foundation and be structurally sound – taking into consideration the physical and emotional safety of the client. It must respond to the specific needs and treatment goals of the client (Smolowe et al., 1999).

Treatment Goal Implementation

As discussed in previous chapters, EAP treatment goals vary depending on the population and purpose. If the team is conducting a workshop or seminar, the goals may be determined by the team and may be general such as teambuilding, communication, or work ethic. This may often be the case when working with groups of any kind – initially the treatment team may set a general goal for the activity and from that specific activity, goals may be discovered and met.

On the other hand, with individual or family therapy, the goals may be very specific and often determined by the client(s). At the onset of therapy, the client(s) should be given the opportunity to verbalize treatment goals for their therapy experience:

- What do they want to accomplish in therapy?
- Why are they here?

With that information, the EAP team begins addressing these issues in activities. All the details of how they handle the issue and/or related issues will surface in the sessions as well. When the team gets preoccupied in trying to simulate a scenario too specifically, they only become boxed in thereby limiting the horses' ability to accurately mirror the dynamics present. Therefore, it is critical for the treatment team to use activities as opportunities while keeping a "curious" mindset about what will transpire as a result.

Setting up the Session

The session setup can be done in various ways. Each EAP team will find a format that works best for them. Some suggestions to having a successful session are as follows:

- Two heads are always better than one – maximize the team approach by discussing the case and goals prior to the session taking place to devise a plan.
- Don't make this harder than it has to be – it is very easy to overanalyze and complicate activities. This can ultimately limit potential outcomes. Keep it simple. The process will be complex enough. If the team makes it too complex, the horse/client dynamic and role may be hindered.
- Be creative and willing to try new activities or make adjustments as needed. For instance, the team explains the next activity to the group. After the group has started working, the team realizes that one team member forgot to say one rule. For the benefit of the clients, do not add and/or change activity rules midstream. At this point, the team needs to go with the flow of what has been laid before the clients already. Let them work with it. Use the process that transpires as an opportunity for learning and growth for the clients.
- Key fact to remember, if a client has a dominant issue that needs addressing (i.e. Anger management), it will surface in the activity, no matter what activity the team gives him/her to work on.
- The activity needs to be viewed as an opportunity to explore the client's journey. Remember the investigatory analogy in Chapter 15, the activity gives you new opportunities for clues to outcomes and/or discovery of puzzle pieces to surface.

Overall, the key to successful facilitation is not worrying that the one opportunity to address an issue will be missed if the activity doesn't go as planned. I have said it many times already; truth is that if the client has an issue that needs addressing, it will come out. The treatment team may be surprised that the issues that come out often are not initially reported but end up being the primary and underlying issues. Remember, if the treatment team finds themselves being rigid about wanting the client and/or session to look one way, they are probably projecting and not trusting the process. For a refresher on addressing this, revisit Chapter 15: Filtering out personal agendas starting on page 229.

Figure 16.1 Temptation Alley is one of the many activities that can look many different ways depending on treatment goals, clients, horses and props available.

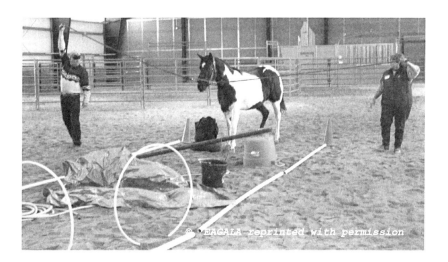

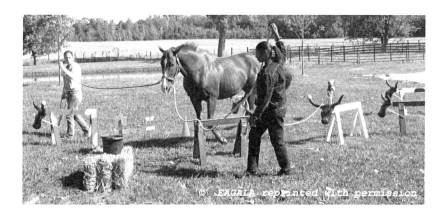

How to Conduct Sessions

Though EAP activities vary dramatically, the process by which the treatment team and client get to that design is fairly uniform. The first step, as stated before, is the needs assessment. It is through this process of gathering and sifting information that the client's agenda becomes clear. Often, the client will prove to have primary and secondary goals (Smolowe et al., 1999). During the EAP activity design phase or working phase, these broad goals are honed, ever-sharpening the focus to produce clarity of purpose. A big-picture outline is then sketched to map out the EAP activity design's flow. Then, a more detailed outline of each session's events is also considered. While some EAP activities need only a loose plan, others require a more detailed design. It is at this point that the EAP treatment team begins to select and customize specific EAP activities around the treatment goals. The deeper the treatment team's knowledge of the client's goals and horses' behavior patterns, the greater their ability to create metaphorical frameworks that will aid in opportunity for each component of the design to be meaningful and memorable for participants (Smolowe et al., 1999). Finally, though an EAP activity may attempt to anticipate and address the client's every need, consideration and problem, it is only a plan or "opportunity for insight." As during construction, so during delivery: unpredictabilities arise, human and/or horse priorities clash – flexibility is essential (Smolowe et al., 1999).

It has been said that conducting an EAP session is "simple but not easy." One of the biggest challenges for many EAP professionals is keeping their mouths shut and silently observing, allowing the clients to progress at their own rate. The most effective EAP team is able to stand back and observe while this process happens without interfering to control the outcome or to rescue the clients. Just as being a good therapist takes discernment and wisdom, being an effective EAP professional requires the same characteristics. EAP professionals must be able to detect when to speak up and when to allow the process to happen. Everything is therapy that takes place during the session from the time the clients arrive until they leave the property. A good EAP treatment team is able to train clients to see the metaphors in the activities just as well as they do.

Processing Activities

The key to EAP activities being generalizable to life is in the processing phase of an activity. The amount of time needed to process will vary with each client, his/her goals, the activity, and the age of the client. Some activities can hold more power if not processed immediately, while others need to be talked about several times throughout the activity while it is happening. Once again, there is always more than one way to effectively process a session. Some common means of processing an activity include discussing the activity and applications, getting clients to write out what they got out of the session and its relevance in their life, and/or videotaping the session and allowing the clients to watch themselves and talk while watching the tape. Depending on what took place during the session keeping therapy goals in mind, the method of processing and length of processing may vary. Nevertheless, as discussed in Chapter 14, the key is that the activity is processed on some level at some time – not necessarily right away.

Facilitators in training often ask, "How do I know when to process and when to let something just sink in without words?" Knowing the best time to stop and process according to Mark Lytle (personal communications, Feb. 2013) depends on "timing, balance and feel," just like horse training. EAGALA (2012) describes this moment in a session as the **peak**, the moment of depth. This is the moment in the session when a level of awareness has been achieved so that the facilitators know to move to a "closure" or break, providing an opportunity for the client to think and process within himself/herself. It can occur at any point in the session, so it is important that facilitators are aware of when "the Peak" point happens. If the facilitators focus too much on this moment verbally, at times, awareness can be replaced with anger, resentment, blaming and defensiveness. Likewise, trying to touch on too many SPUD's or over-processing can be overwhelming and confusing. Pace the sessions and remember that if it is truly important, the issues will continue to surface in the next session. Peaks are sometimes obvious but most often very subtle. Observing the horses and being attuned to the client's nonverbal cues are central to recognizing Peaks (EAGALA, 2012). Randy Mandrell (personal communications, 2011) compares this Peak moment as "the moment to release pressure." He compares this process to training horses. When training a horse, the trainer adds pressure until the horse has a moment of optimal learning, then releases the pressure. The horse then learns from this moment and is able to progress from there in the next training session. Mandrell (2011) believes that this is the same process that is occurring with the client. The horse activity and observations create pressure and once the client reaches that moment of depth, or "awareness," release the pressure by stopping the activity, discussing, and/or not talking, whichever will release the pressure for that client in the moment. This is a balance or dance, a skill that improves with practice.

Some of the questions that are often asked during a processing session may include:

> - What were your thoughts and feelings during this activity?
> - How did the horses respond in this activity? What relevance does that hold for you?
> - In what ways were your behaviors/responses like your responses in life?
> - What did you learn from this activity about yourself? About others?

Allotting Adequate Time for Activities

"How much time will this activity take?" is always a difficult question to answer yet one frequently asked by professionals and clients alike. This depends on so many factors that are out of the EAP team's control. Therefore, most EAP professionals set a session time limit just like they would in a traditional therapy format. If the activity does not get done in that amount of time, that is okay. The main objective and goal in an EAP session is not to complete the activity necessarily, but to observe and discuss the process of how the clients work toward the completion of the activity. Frequently, an activity takes several sessions before being completed. The activity can be a metaphor within itself representing the problems that brought them to therapy. They will not get over their issues in one session, just as they may not be able to complete the activity at hand in one session. Success in EAP is not defined by completing the activity but in the process of how the clients work through the difficult situations.

On the flip side, many EAP professionals fear that if the clients complete the activity really quickly, they will not have anything to process. They worry and question, "What will we do with the rest of the session time?" Remarkably, five minutes worth of activity can still be loaded with information to process. Do not underestimate the significance of an activity that is completed quickly. This too is valuable information to process. The fact that they were prompt is something to process within itself: What does that say about them? What contributed to their prompt completion? How did the horse impact this? After processing the activity, you have a few choices to consider: end the session early, duplicate the same activity with a different horse and get a different response, or move on to another activity. They may have successfully addressed this issue and may be ready to move on. The treatment team must make this decision based on the needs of the clients in relation to their progress and treatment goals, considering the previous discussion regarding peak and the pressure/release concept. The main question to ask as a treatment team is "Has the client peaked? Does the treatment team need to release pressure?"

Documenting Progress

Young (1992) describes a five-part model for the progression of counseling that is also present in Equine-Assisted Psychotherapy. This progression in EAP begins with the initial relationship-building issues through assessment, treatment planning, implementing EAP activities to address issues, and finally concluding with evaluation. **Evaluation** is the process of reviewing and re-planning counseling goals. Termination may soon follow the evaluation stage, as a result of therapeutic gains, or a client may indicate that new issues have arisen (Young, 1992). One key issue related to the evaluation phase is client progress notes, which are an integral part of helping clients achieve treatment goals. Documenting progress using case notes or progress notes is an activity almost universally despised by clinicians. Still, most recognize it as an important legal necessity and is a useful record of the client's progress over time (Piazza & Baruth, 1990). Clearly, the EAP format is no exception.

One example of a format presented by Young (1992) often used by mental health professionals for documenting case notes that is easily converted for EAP professionals is the REPLAN system. REPLAN is an acronym for: **R**elationship, **E**fficacy & self-esteem, **P**racticing new behaviors, **L**owering or rising emotional arousal, **A**ctivating expectations and motivation, and **N**ew learning experiences and changing perceptions. The REPLAN system is considered easy to use because, rather than being confronted with a blank space, the therapist is asked to answer specific questions about the treatment goals:

- What progress was made since the last session?
- What important crises changes have occurred in the client's life or mental status since the last session?
- What progress was made toward each client goal in today's session?
- What plans, activities, homework, or referrals were made today?
- When should the client's goals be reviewed?

The REPLAN record (Tables 16.1 and Table 16.2) adapted from Young (1992) begins by listing previously agreed-upon client goals expressed in the treatment plan. The first step for the EAP professionals is to briefly note any changes or progress on goals reported by the client since the last session. Next, the EAP professional records any new information – a job change, a change in relationships, changes in behavior, or changes in client's mental status. Third, the therapist documents the strategies employed to achieve counseling goals during the session. This is where the EAP activity will be described. Fourth, the EAP professionals indicate what plans were agreed upon for homework, practice, and outside referrals. The REPLAN system allows new goals to be added or removed from consideration at each session.

TABLE 16.1 REPLAN Counseling Record and Case Notes: Format #1

Client Name:_____   Session No. _____   Date_____

Goal No.	Therapy Goals	Any Progress/Changes in Mental Status	Activity Directed Toward Goals	Homework/ Referrals/ Plans

Counselor Signature_____

Horse Professional Signature_____

REPLAN Date _____

TABLE 16.2 REPLAN Counseling Record and Case Notes: Format #2.

Client Name _____ Session No. _____
Date _____
Therapy Goals:
1.
2.
3

Any Progress in Goals Since Last Session
1.
2.
3.

New Information (Changes in client's situation or mental status)

EAP Activity During This Session:
Goal 1:
Goal 2:
Goal 3:

Homework Assignments, Referrals, and Plans
Goal   Plan
1.
2.
3.

Counselor Signature:_____

Horse Professional Signature:_____

REPLAN date _____

The numbering system in the progress notes always refers to the same goal from the therapy goals at the top of the form. Consequently, there is no need to rewrite the description of the goal in later portions of the notes (Young, 1992). Tables 16.1 and 16.2 demonstrate two frequently used formats to the REPLAN system. Either variation is adequate for EAP as well; the difference is merely preference in organizational structure.

CHAPTER 16

EAGALA (2006) developed and trademarked a format that is unique to the model that focuses on the SPUD's discussed in Chapter 14. Table 16.3 shows this format which focuses on the shifts, patterns, unique moments, discrepancies, and self-awareness and can be adapted to incorporate specific treatment goals to each observation. The triangle indicates the top 3 spuds that lead up to the peak moment in the session. The specific use of the case notes may influence the format you choose. The EAGALA format focuses more on non-verbal observations while the REPLAN format focuses more on verbal feedback. All formats have pros and cons, so the appropriateness of format will depend of treatment plan needs and purpose.

TABLE 16.3 SPUD's Format

Treatment Team Members: _____
Date of Session: _____
Time length of Session: _____ Session # for this client or group: _____
  ❑ Family   Number involved: _____
  ❑ Individual M or F   Age: _____

SPUD'S

What did you see as the peak?

S –

P –

U –   3.

D –
                    2.

'S
            1.

Themes (for treatment planning and planning next session) –

© *EAGALA reprinted with permission*

There is a discussion within the field about case note requirements for the horse professional in the EAP team. Do they need to be writing case notes as well? Some EAP horse professionals are signing the therapist's progress notes, while others are not signing any paperwork at all. Many professionals in the field believe that the horse professional should be operating under the same legal obligations and ethics as the therapists in all areas including case notes. Other professionals have recommended that horse professionals take progress notes but from a different perspective than the therapist. These professionals are not against the horse professional signing off on the therapist's case notes, but many believe that the horse professional's main duty in documentation is to keep records on the horses and their behaviors. Within this perspective, the horse professional should keep a file on each horse, just as therapists keep client files. In each file, the horse professional should have health records and care charts. Also, there should be a brief progress note for every session the horse is involved in indicating activity, behavior, patterns, and/or exceptions to patterns. Incident reports would be kept in these files as well. These professionals argue this practice only increases the level of professionalism while providing liability protection for the EAP team regarding their equine partners.

No matter what approach you take in record keeping, remember that EAP is professional counseling and must follow all ethical and legal guidelines for your state and licensing governing body. Facilitating an EAP activity includes more than what transpires in the arena. Success in this model includes much preparation and follow through as a team behind the scenes.

Topics of Discussion:

1. You have a teenage client who has been disrespecting his parents and teachers. He is failing all his classes and skipping school. For today's activity, you take him out to a very large pasture and ask him to catch and halter the horse. (Note to team: this horse is EXTREMELY hard to catch and you are planning on this taking the entire session). The client walks out in the pasture and the horse runs up to him. He has the horse

CHAPTER 16

haltered within the first 5 minutes of the session. What do you do with the rest of your time? Discuss your plan.

2. *Practice writing a progress note on the above session scenario using the REPLAN system design or SPUD design. Discuss your preference in format and explain.*

3. *Several perspectives were presented about whether or not horse professionals should write case notes. What are your thoughts on this discussion? Explain your position.*

4. *What do you foresee will be the most challenging aspect of conducting an EAP session for you? Explain.*

Chapter Notes

Chapter Notes

17 ASSESSMENT AND EVALUATION

Objectives:
- **Discuss the impact assessment has in therapy**
- **Demonstrate information gathering tools**
- **Explore various evaluation perspectives**
- **Emphasize the role professional evaluation has on outcome**
- **Evaluate the ethical and clinical implications of professional assessment**

This chapter will discuss further the importance of assessment and evaluation in the EAP therapeutic process. It will explore several examples of intake procedures and evaluation measures. By the end of this chapter, the treatment team should grasp the significance of assessment and evaluation of the client, the program, and the treatment team. This process is a continuous one and should be reviewed and explored on a regular basis. As an EAP professional, one should always be looking to grow and improve.

The Importance of Assessment

As previously mentioned in this book, assessment is essential to the progress of all therapy processes. Whether traditional or nontraditional, the style of assessment is up to the therapy professional. In Equine-Assisted Psychotherapy, the assessment and evaluation processes can be done either in the arena using the horses or in the office using the more traditional talk format to gather information, or a combination of the two.

One advantage to using the horses in the information gathering phase of therapy is that the information received tends to be more authentic and to the point. Because of the non-threatening and unintrusive approach of the horses, the client is more open with true thoughts and feelings; therefore, the issues surface more quickly. In the office, clients often have a difficult time putting their thoughts and feelings into words, and/or they are concerned about what the therapist will think about them at this point. The horse can help to break these barriers and speeds up the building rapport stage of the therapy process.

Some therapists come from the therapeutic orientation that promotes a very detailed and comprehensive description up front about a client's issues and past history, while most EAP professionals and therapists tend to move away from this approach the longer they do this work. In the assessment phase of EAP, it is only necessary to know generally what the core issues are to be addressed. The details will come out in the process in a way that aids the client in working through them. In EAP, assessment and evaluation are a continuous process and are present from the onset to termination with a client.

In the first few sessions, the treatment team is not only assessing the client with regards to issues that need to be addressed but also evaluating their client's level of comfort and knowledge about horses. All aspects are important components of the initial stage of EAP. This information gathered, during the beginning exposure with the horses, helps the horse professional better match the client to a horse and/or activity for the sessions to come. This lets the team know how quickly to progress in the process of interaction with the horses. Remember, this information is also metaphorical for the client's interactions with relationships in life. Therefore, the team needs to be evaluating the client's response to this experience on two levels - both the literal and the figurative.

Techniques and Procedures

There are many techniques and procedures for gathering information in the client assessment process. A sample procedure includes assessment and information gathering prior to the client's arrival to the barn for therapy – phone intake, intake form to be completed upon arrival, and case notes for further information. Tables 17.1 through 17.3 are sample intake paperwork forms that can be very beneficial to gathering information for initial assessment. This format is not to be copied in its entirety without modifications according to your state regulations and licensing procedures.

CHAPTER 17

Table 17.1 – Sample EAP Intake Inventory

CLIENT INFORMATION	FAMILY/SPOUSE INFORMATION

Name:_____ Sex: M F
Address: _____
City, State, Zip: _____
Home Phone: _____
Employer: _____
Business Phone: _____
SS#: _____ DOB_____
Age____
Married   Remarried   Single
   Engaged   Widowed
     Separated   Divorced
 	
Court Involvement: _____
Other agencies involved: _____
	Spouse / Parent: _____
	Address: _____
	City, State, Zip: _____
	Home Phone: _____
	Employer: _____
	Business Phone: _____
	SS#:_____ DOB_____ Age____
	
	Married Remarried Single
	   Engaged Widowed
	     Separated Divorced

Education 1 2 3 4 5 6 7 8 9 10 11 12 13 14 15 16 17+
Other (list types and years) _____

Information on children—
Name:	Age:	Sex:	Living:		School Grade:
_____	_____	M F	In Home	Out of Home	_____
_____	_____	M F	In Home	Out of Home	_____
_____	_____	M F	In Home	Out of Home	_____
_____	_____	M F	In Home	Out of Home	_____
_____	_____	M F	In Home	Out of Home	_____

PARENTAL CONSENT
MUST BE COMPLETED FOR ALL CLIENTS UNDER AGE OF 18+
I, legal guardian, give my authorization for EAP SERVICES to counsel with the above-mentioned minor.
Signature: _____ Date: _____

HEALTH
How would you rate your physical health?   Very Good   Good   Average   Poor
If you are presently taking any medication please list medication: _____
For what condition? _____ Medical Doctor: _____
Name of referring physician, if any: _____

COUNSELING DATA
How did you hear about EAP SERVICES?
Friend   Family Member   Phone Book   Brochure   Other _____
Have you ever been seen or treated by a psychiatrist, counselor, or therapist Yes, How long?_____   No
Please state in a few sentences the major counseling need you have at this time _____
_____
_____
_____

Table 17.2 – Sample EAP Disclosure and Consent Form

DISCLOSURE AND CONSENT STATEMENT

The following is to inform you of the policies and therapeutic practices of EAP SERVICES. Please read this information carefully. If you have any questions please feel free to discuss this with your therapist.

CLINICAL AND THERAPIST INFORMATION

A primary commitment of EAP SERVICES is to provide you with quality counseling services. However, no counselor can guarantee that counseling services will be effective for you. This statement is intended to convey pertinent information regarding our services, allowing you to make choices based on correct information. All our therapists have either Masters or Doctoral level degrees and work in partnership with an EAGALA certified horse professional. Therapists are either licensed by the State as Professional Counselors, or they are working toward licensure under an approved supervisor. We endeavor to maintain a high level of competence and we adhere to professional, legal, and moral standards. Equine-Assisted Psychotherapy is a team approach to counseling with a therapist, horse professional, and a horse. We seek to integrate the emotional, spiritual, physical, relational, and mental elements in the counseling process. A variety of techniques and approaches are used. If you have any further questions regarding your therapist's training or professional approach, please feel free to ask your therapist.

APPOINTMENT AND FEE POLICY

I. The normal fee for our services is $XXX per session depending on treatment design. Fees must be paid out of pocket. We are not set up to bill insurance directly. All those who have insurance to assist with this fee are expected to handle payment for services and bill their insurance company themselves. We are willing to provide receipts needed to do so. It is your responsibility to see that the fee is covered. If you will be filing on your insurance, it is IMPORTANT that you realize we must assign a diagnosis, and that diagnosis will permanently be on your medical record. Payment is due at the time services are rendered.

II. If you are unable to keep your appointment, please give a 24-hour notice so that we may utilize the time to assist someone else. Unless there is an extreme emergency, we will charge you one half of your fee if a 24-hour notice is not given and the full fee for missed appointments with no notice. The fees are to be paid by the next appointment. I have read and understand the appointment and fee policy. _____ (initial).

CONFIDENTIALITY INFORMATION

I. Content obtained in the counseling sessions will be handled professionally and confidentially. This information will be used by your therapist, the horse professional, and the supervisor for your therapeutic benefit. If for treatment purposes, we need information from another party, we will ask you to sign a Release of Information Form.

II. To further maximize the benefits of therapy activities and to assess these benefits, you may be asked to complete a pre-test before starting therapy and post-test after completion of therapy. The data collected will be used to improve therapy services for others in the future and to provide data needed in grant applications. No personal information will be disclosed in these findings.

CHAPTER 17

Table 17.2 – Sample EAP Disclosure and Consent Form continues…

III. Confidentiality is forfeited for any of the following:
   A. If you pose serious physical danger to yourself or another person
   B. If you disclose that you or another person has physically or sexually abused or molested a child or an incompetent or disabled person.
   C. If you disclose that a child, an incompetent or disabled person is suffering from neglect.
   D. Defense of claims brought by client against the therapist and/or horse professional of EAP SERVICES.
   E. Reporting to relevant agencies such as court and insurance co. as may be ordered by the Court system or for third party payment
   F. If you disclose that you have committed a crime.

If any of A-F apply immediate action must be taken. I have read and understand the Confidentiality Information. _____(Initial).

CONSENT TO TREATMENT

After thoroughly reading, understanding and receiving a copy of the above information, I give my consent to treatment (including assessment and therapy) to EAP Services. I have read and understand the policies and information stated above.

Signature _____   Date _____

In addition to assessment gathering tools and paperwork, it is vital for the treatment team to maintain adequate case notes on each client and session. Not only is this mandatory by licensing agencies but also good practice for the professional to work by. Even though the atmosphere of therapy in EAP is much more relaxed than many therapists' offices, the standards and quality should not be jeopardized. All procedures improve professional practice and show responsible practice if ever questioned by a court at law.

ASSESSMENT AND EVALUATION

Table 17.3 -- Registration and Release Form

REGISTRATION:

Client:_____ Date of Birth:_____ Age:_____
Street:_____
City/State:_____ Zip Code:_____
Home #:_____ Work #:_____ Emergency #:_____
Parent or Legal Guardian Name(s):_____
Home #:_____ Work #:_____ Emergency #:_____
School Attending:_____ Grade:_____
Court Involvement:_____ On Probation:_____
Other Agencies involved with client:_____

CONSENT AND WAIVER OF LIABILITY:

I, _____, hereby request that the client named above be accepted into the equine-assisted psychotherapy program operated by EAP SERVICES. I acknowledge that EAP SERVICES Personnel have fully explained to me the scope of the equine-assisted psychotherapy (EAP) program, including the potential for injury which can occur from riding horses, caring for horses or being involved in therapeutic activities that include horses. Because of the potential benefits of the EAP program, I hereby waive any claim which I or the client may have against EAP SERVICES, officers, employees, volunteer, or contract personnel arising out of any injury which the client may sustain while involved in the EAP program, unless caused by the willful misconduct or gross negligence of EAP SERVICES, its employees, officers, volunteer, or contract personnel.

The undersigned assumes the unavoidable risks inherent in all horse-related activities, including but not limited to bodily injury and physical harm to horse, rider and spectator. In consideration, therefore, for the privilege of riding and/or working and/or participating in activities around horses with EAP SERVICES.

_____, the undersigned does hereby agree to hold harmless and indemnify EAP SERVICES, its employees, officers, volunteers, and contract personnel, and further release them from any liability or responsibility for accident, damage, injury or illness to the Undersigned or to any horse owned by the Undersigned or to any family member or spectator accompanying the Undersigned on the premises.

I have read this release.

Signature of client	Date
Signature of Parent or Guardian	Date
Signature of therapist	Date

Table 17.4 -- Sample Medical History/ Physician Release

Name: _____
Date of Birth: _____
Address: _____
Name of Parent/Guardian: _____
Tetnus Shot: Yes / No Date: _____ Height: _____ Weight: _____
Medications taking: _____

Please indicate if client has a problem and/or surgeries in any of the following areas by checking yes or no. If yes, please comment, using back of form if necessary.

AREAS	YES	NO	COMMENTS
Auditory			
Visual			
Speech			
Cardiac			
Circulatory (inc. Hemophilia)			
Pulmonary			
Neurological			
Muscular			
Orthopedic (incl. Spinal/Joint Abnormalities)			
Allergies (incl. Asthma)			
Learning Disability			
Mental Impairment			
Psychological Impairment (incl. Behavioral)			
Diabetes (note restrictions if any)			
Other:			

PHYSICIAN MUST SIGN BELOW FOR ALL CLIENTS

In my opinion, this patient can participate in supervised equestrian activities.
Physician's Signature: _____
Physician's Name (please print): _____
Address/City/Zip: _____
Phone: ( ) _____ Date: _____

Signature of Parent or legal guardian: _____

In addition to assessment gathering tools and paperwork, it is vital for the treatment team to maintain adequate case notes on each client and session. Not only is this mandatory by licensing agencies but also good practice for the professional to work by. Even though the atmosphere of therapy in EAP is much more relaxed than many therapists' offices, the standards and quality should not be jeopardized. EAP therapists and horse professionals alike should maintain notes on clients. Whether the team does the notes together or separately is up to the team's discretion. Many programs require horse professionals to document horses' behaviors during therapy along with medical, feeding, and hoof care documentation on each therapy horse. All procedures improve professional practice and show responsible practice if ever questioned by a court at law. Table 17.4 gives an example of a medical history form used by many EAP professionals in this field. Again, this form must be adapted before use to meet the standards of your licensing agency and state requirements.

Professional Assessment and Evaluation

Professional assessment is vital to the success of therapy and business. The therapist, as well as horse professional, needs to find some sort of accountability system to stay sharp and ensure that personal issues do not interfere with therapy. As discussed many times in this book, countertransference is a legitimate concern in this type of therapy and must be acknowledged.

According to Corey, Corey, and Callanan (1998), a primary issue in the helping professions is the role of the counselor *as a person* in the therapeutic relationship. Because EAP professionals are asking clients to look honestly at themselves and to choose how they want to change, EAP professionals must open their own lives to the same scrutiny. They should repeatedly ask themselves these questions: *"What makes me think I am capable of helping anyone? What do I personally have to offer others who are struggling to find their way? Am I doing in my own life what I urge others to do?"*

Counselors and psychotherapists usually acquire an extensive theoretical and practical knowledge as a basis for their practice. But they also bring their human qualities and their life experiences to every therapeutic session. EAP professionals can be well versed in psychological theory, EAP philosophy, horse psychology, and diagnostic and interviewing skills and still be ineffective helpers. If EAP professionals are to promote growth and change in their clients, they must be willing to promote growth in their own lives. This willingness to live in accordance with what they teach is what makes an EAP professional a "therapeutic person." If EAP professionals are stagnant themselves, it is doubtful that they can inspire clients to make life-affirming choices. Ethical problems can arise when EAP professionals are unable to carry out this modeling role, which is critical in encouraging clients to change.

It is difficult to talk about the EAP professional *as a professional* without considering personal qualities. An EAP professional's beliefs, personal attributes, and ways of living inevitably influences the way s/he functions as a professional. EAP professionals often take up problems that are closely linked to their personal lives: self-awareness and the influence of the EAP professional's personality and needs, transference and counter transference, job stress, and the challenge of remaining vital both personally and professionally. Corey, Corey, and Callanan (1998) devised the following self-inventory on Table 17.5 that can help the treatment team identify and clarify your attitudes and beliefs about the issues around professional assessment. They suggest that one keep in mind that the "right" answer is the one that best expresses your thoughts at the time. Corey, Corey, and Callanan (1998) suggest that each team member complete the inventory before reading this section; then, after reading the chapter, retake the inventory to see whether positions have changed in any way.

Table 17.5 -- Self-Inventory

Directions: For each statement, indicate the response that most closely identifies your beliefs and attitudes. Use the following code:

    5 = I *strongly agree* with this statement
    4 = I *agree* with this statement
    3 = I am *undecided* about this statement
    2 = I *disagree* with this statement
    1 = I *strongly disagree* with this statement

___ 1. Unless EAP professionals have a high degree of self-awareness, there is a real danger that they will use their clients to satisfy their own needs.
___ 2. Before EAP professionals begin to practice, they should be free of personal problems and conflicts
___ 3. EAP professionals should be required to undergo their own therapy before they are licensed or certified to practice.
___ 4. EAP professionals who satisfy their needs through their work are behaving unethically.
___ 5. Many EAP professionals face a high risk of burnout because of the demands of their jobs.
___ 6. EAP professionals who know themselves can avoid experiencing over identification with their clients.
___ 7. Strong feelings about a client are a sign that the EAP professional needs further therapy.
___ 8. Feelings of anxiety in a beginning EAP professional indicate unsuitability for the EAP profession.
___ 9. A competent EAP professional can work with any client.
___ 10. I fear that I'll have difficulty challenging my clients.
___ 11. An EAP professional will avoid getting involved socially with clients or counseling friends.
___ 12. A major fear of mine is that I'll make mistakes and seriously hurt a client.
___ 13. Real therapy does not occur unless a transference relationship is developed.
___ 14. I think it is important to adapt my therapeutic techniques and approaches to the cultural background of my clients.
___ 15. An experienced and competent EAP professional should not need either periodic or ongoing personal psychotherapy.

Personal Needs of EAP Professionals

The rewards of practicing EAP are many, but one of the most significant is the joy of seeing clients move from being victims to assuming control over their lives. Treatment teams can achieve this reward only if they avoid abusing their influence and maintain a keen awareness of their role as facilitators of others' growth. As the treatment team considers their own needs and influences on their work as an EAP professional, they both might ask themself the following questions adapted from Corey, Corey, and Callanan (1998):

- ➤ How can I know when I'm working for the client's benefit and when I'm working for my own benefit?
- ➤ How much might I depend on clients to tell me how good I am as a person or as an EAP professional? Am I able to appreciate myself, or do I depend primarily on others to validate my worth and the value of my work?
- ➤ Do I always feel inadequate when clients don't make progress? If so, how could my attitude and feelings of inadequacy adversely affect my work with clients?

Personal Therapy for EAP Professionals

It is debated in the field whether all therapists should be involved in personal counseling themselves to be effective facilitators. This same question can be posed for those professionals in the field of EAP. Whether you believe this to be true or not, the following questions adapted from Corey, Corey, and Callanan (1998) should be considered by all members of the treatment team. Personal therapy for EAP professionals raises questions such as:

- ➤ How am I feeling about my own values as an EAP professional?
- ➤ Do I like my relationship with my client?
- ➤ What reactions are being evoked in me as I work with this client?
- ➤ What kind of self-exploration have I engaged in prior to or during my training?
- ➤ How open am I to looking at personal characteristics that could be either strengths or limitations as an EAP professional?
- ➤ What am I willing to do to work through personal problems I have at this time?

Transference: The "Unreal" Relationship in Therapy

As defined previously in this book, transference is the process whereby clients project onto their treatment team past feelings or attitudes they had toward significant people in their lives (Corey, Corey, and Callanan, 1998).

Watkins (1983) identified five transference patterns in counseling and psychotherapy. The following patterns are adapted from his original list:

1. *EAP professional as ideal.* The client sees the EAP professionals as perfect people who do everything right.
2. *EAP professional as seer.* Clients view the EAP professional as an expert, all-knowing.
3. *EAP professional as nurturer.* Some clients look to the EAP professionals for nurturing and feeding, as a small child would.
4. *EAP professional as frustrator.* The client is defensive, cautious, and guarded and is constantly testing the EAP professionals.
5. *EAP professional as nonentity.* In this form of transference, the client regards the EAP professionals as inanimate figures without needs, desires, wishes, or problems.

Countertransference: Ethical and Clinical Implications

As previously discussed and explored in this book, countertransference can be considered, in the broad sense, as any projections by a member of the treatment team that can potentially get in the way of helping a client (Corey, Corey, and Callanan, 1998).

Countertransference can show itself in many ways. Adapted from Corey, Corey, and Callanan (1998), each example in the following list presents an ethical issue because the EAP professional's effective work is obstructed by countertransference reactions:

1. *Being overprotective with a client* can reflect an EAP professional's deep fears.

   ❖ Are you aware of reacting to certain types of people in overprotective ways? If so, what might this behavior reveal about you?
   ❖ Do you find that you are able to allow others to experience their pain or do you have a tendency to want to take their pain away quickly?

2. *Treating clients in a benign* way may stem from an EAP professional's fear of the client's anger.

   ❖ Do you ever find yourself saying things to guard against another's anger?
   ❖ What might you say or do if you became aware that your exchanges with a client were primarily superficial?

3. *Rejecting a client* may be based on the EAP professional's perception of the client as needy and dependent.

   ❖ Do you find yourself wanting to create distance from certain types of people?
   ❖ What can you learn about yourself by looking at those people whom you are likely to reject?

4. *Needing constant reinforcement and approval* can be a reflection of countertransference. Just as clients may develop an excessive need to please their EAP professionals to feel liked and valued, EAP professionals may have an inordinate need to be reassured of their effectiveness.

> - ❖ Do you need to have the approval of your clients? How willing are you to confront them even at the risk of being disliked?
> - ❖ What is your style of confronting a client? Do you tend to confront certain kinds of clients more frequently and/or assertively than others? What does this behavior tell you about yourself as an EAP professional?

5. *Seeing yourself in your clients* is another form of countertransference. This is not to say that feeling close to a client and identifying with that person's struggle is necessarily countertransference. They become so lost in a client's world that they are unable to distinguish their own feelings.

> - ❖ Have you ever found yourself so much in sympathy with others that you could no longer be of help to them? What would you do if you felt this way about a client?
> - ❖ From an awareness of your own dynamics, list some personal traits of clients that would be most likely to elicit over identification on your part.

6. *Developing sexual or romantic feelings* toward a client exploits the vulnerable position of the client.

> - ❖ What would you do if you experienced intense sexual feelings toward a client?
> - ❖ How would you know if your sexual attraction to a client was countertransference or not?

7. *Giving advice compulsively* can easily be encouraged by clients who seek immediate answers to ease their suffering.

> - ❖ Do you ever find yourself giving advice? What do you think you gain from it? In what ways might the advice you give to clients represent advice that you could give yourself?
> - ❖ Are there ever times when advice is warranted? If so, when?

8. *Desiring a social relationship with clients* may stem from countertransference, especially if it is acted on while therapy is taking place.

> ❖ If I establish a social relationship with certain clients, will I be as inclined to confront them in therapy as I would be otherwise?
> ❖ Will my own needs for preserving these friendships interfere with my therapeutic activities and defeat the purpose of therapy?
> ❖ Am I sensitive to being called a "cold professional," even though I may strive to be real and straightforward in the therapeutic situation?
> ❖ Why am I inclined to form friendships with clients? Does this practice serve my own or my clients' best interests?

Stress in the EAP Profession

Bennett, Bryant, VandenBos, and Greenwood (1990) raise the following questions that can help you assess the impact of stress on one both personally and professionally. Consider the following questions when evaluating how stress is affecting professionalism:

> ➤ Do you ignore your problems out of fear?
> ➤ Have you learned techniques for managing stress, such as time management and relaxation training?
> ➤ Are you able to take care of your personal needs?
> ➤ Are you aware of the signs and symptoms warning you that you are in trouble?
> ➤ Do you listen to your family, friends, and colleagues when they tell you that stress is getting the better of you?
> ➤ Do you consider seeking help when you notice you are exhibiting signs of stress?

Stress is related to irrational beliefs that many EAP professionals hold. Practitioners with exceptionally high goals or perfectionist strivings related to helping others often report a high level of stress (Corey, Corey, Callanan, 1998). Deutsch (1984) gives the following examples of the three most stressful beliefs, all of which pertain to doing perfect work with clients:

1. "I should always work at my peak level of enthusiasm and competence."
2. "I should be able to cope with any client emergency that arises."
3. "I should be able to help every client."

According to Corey, Corey, & Callanan (1998), some other irrational beliefs that lead to stress are:

- "When a client does not make progress, it is my fault."
- "I should not take off time from work when I know that a particular client needs me."
- "My job is my life."
- "I should be a model of mental health."
- "I should be 'on call' at all times."
- "A client's needs always come before my own."
- "I am the most important person in my client's life."
- "I am responsible for my client's behavior."
- "I have the power to control my client's life."

It is interesting to note that these beliefs are related to the basic reasons many people choose the helping professions. The needs of helpers are to be needed by others, to feel important, to have an impact on the lives of others, to have the power to control others, and to be significant. When helpers are able to do these things successfully, they are likely to feel that they are making a significant difference in the lives of their clients. When they feel that they are not making a difference and are not reaching clients, stress affects them more dramatically. Beliefs that create stress are those that goad the EAP professional to constantly produce at maximum levels, a pace that eventually leads to burnout.

EAP Professional Impairment

Corey, Corey, & Callanan (1998) pose an important question to consider, *"What can you do not only to prevent yourself from becoming an impaired professional but also to become committed to promoting your own wellness from holistic perspective?"* If needing to explore this further go back to Chapter 15, Table 15.3; these questions can help one work through filtering self-awareness through to a processing stage (p. 230).

Some questions Benningfield (1994) offers for this self-assessment include:

> - Is my personal life satisfying and rewarding? Are my relationships what I want them to be?
> - To what degree am I taking care of myself, both physically and emotionally?
> - Would I be willing for other therapists I respect to know about my professional conduct and decisions? Am I willing to express my vulnerabilities through consultation or peer supervision?
> - Can I acknowledge and disclose my mistakes? Am I willing to acknowledge my limitations in my professional role?
> - Am I generally consistent in my practice?
> - Do I think or fantasize about a relationship that goes beyond being a professional with some clients or students?
> - Do I talk about subjects in therapy that are not related to clients' concerns?

Program Assessment – Technique and Process

In addition to personal assessment and evaluation, evaluating and assessing the success of outcomes and services is important. As discussed previously in this book, there are not many statistics available to show the long term benefits and/or success of using horses in psychotherapy to date. Therefore, it is important to the future of one's practice and the field of EAP as a whole to find some form of evaluating outcomes and client's thoughts/feelings about services rendered. Table 17.6 is a sample program and/or therapy evaluation form that can help with program evaluation and data collection for research statistics.

ASSESSMENT AND EVALUATION

Table 17.6 -- Equine-Assisted Psychotherapy Evaluation Form

Number of Sessions Attended: _____
Presenting Problem?
_____
_____

Severity of Problem at onset of counseling vs. upon termination:
Beginning Therapy:
As bad as it can get   Ideal Life
1   2   3   4   5   6   7   8   9   10

Termination of Therapy:
As bad as it can get   Ideal Life
1   2   3   4   5   6   7   8   9   10

Was there a particular session you found more helpful than others? Please explain.
_____
_____

What did you enjoy most of the sessions you attended? What did you enjoy least of the sessions you attended?
_____
_____

Please circle one number for each question. Did you feel you learned skills to help you in the area of:

	Did learn				Did not learn
*communication	1	2	3	4	5
*problem solving	1	2	3	4	5
*stress management	1	2	3	4	5
*anger management	1	2	3	4	5
*boundaries	1	2	3	4	5
*respect for self and others	1	2	3	4	5
*relationships	1	2	3	4	5
*trust	1	2	3	4	5
*other: _____	1	2	3	4	5

What were you hoping to learn from the Equine-Assisted Psychotherapy experience?
_____
_____

Table 17.6 -- Equine-Assisted Psychotherapy Evaluation Form continues….

What specific suggestions would you have for future programs and sessions?
_____
_____
_____

Where did you hear about EAP Services?
       ____ Past Participant
       ____ Radio
       ____ TV
       ____ Newspaper
       ____ Friend
       ____ Family
       ____ Counselor
       ____ Agency: _____
       ____ Other: _____

What ideas do you have for additional growth for you and/or your family, organization, or group?
_____
_____
_____

Thank you for your participation!

Conclusion

Heady (2003, May/June) explains that ethics are merely a judgment of "right and wrong" within a scope of practice. Nevertheless, whether you are the therapist or horse professional part of the EAP treatment team, the team abides by the code of ethics established by the American Counseling Association. Within that code, the treatment team agrees to practice within the therapist's scope of practice. Ethically, one should work in areas where he/she has training, experience, and/or documented competency.

Heady (2003, May/June) continues by emphasizing that activity labeled therapy or therapeutic such as Equine-Assisted Psychotherapy, should actually be provided as therapy, with the therapist present. If as a horseperson, one chooses to give horsemanship lessons or experiences that are well meaning and helpful to at-risk individuals, one still needs to call it what it is -- horsemanship or experiential interactions-- not "therapy or therapeutic." In conclusion, the best way to protect the clients, the equine professional, the mental health professional, the horses, and the field of Equine Assisted Psychotherapy is to practice with the expertise of both the mental health field and the equine world in the same arena at the same time (Heady, 2003, May/June).

The long term benefits of Equine-Assisted Psychotherapy greatly depend on the questions asked by the treatment team. Assessment and evaluation of the client, professionals, and programs are no different. Questioning the process is one of the keys to success of this field. Questioning the process never ends – always assess and always evaluate, being flexible to change and grow it goes. A few last questions to ask before concluding this chapter on assessment and evaluation include:

> ➤ What personal needs of yours will be met by counseling others?
> ➤ To what degree might your needs get in the way of your work with clients?
> ➤ How can you recognize and meet your needs – which are a real part of you, without having them interfere with your work with others? (Corey, Corey, and Callanan, 1998).

After reading this book in its entirety, one should grasp a rather complete picture of the most significant components involved in the theory and practice of Equine-Assisted Psychotherapy. Nevertheless, the information has not near the comprehension without actually stepping into an arena with the horses and experiencing EAP for oneself.

Topics of Discussion:

1. Complete the self-inventory and compare your responses prior to reading the chapter versus after reading the chapter. Explain any differences.

2. Throughout the chapter, there are many questions posed regarding professional assessment and evaluation. Explain your answers to each of these questions.

3. At the very end of the chapter, there are three final questions to ask yourself. Defend your response to these questions.

4. After taking the self-inventory and answering the many questions regarding personal assessment, describe your level of professionalism on a scale of 1 to 10. (10 represents highest level of professionalism while 1 would be completely lacking). Explain the impacts this could pose to your EAP sessions and/or clients.

Chapter Notes

Chapter Notes

APPENDIX

Sample Activities

    Group – Raging River

    Family – Extended Appendages

    Individual – My World

EAP Certification information

Code of Ethics

Bibliography

GROUP ACTIVITY

Raging River

Type: Group; Professionalism in EAP teams

Group size: 6 – 12 participants

Time frame: 45 min -1 hour minutes depending on group size

Materials:
    2-3 horses (to represent "clients")
    2-3 halters & lead ropes
    2 poles (to mark the shores)
    additional random props to represent tools and strengths as professionals such as:
- poles
- buckets with feed in it
- shovel
- cones
- bucket of water
- barrel
- noodles
- hay
- chair
- Sticky labels and markers to label the assets

Goals:
- Identify strengths and growth areas within EAP professionals
- Emphasize importance of health and wellness within EAP team
- Demonstrate impact self-awareness has in improving the ethics of a professional

Setup:
    Set 2 poles on ground approximately 30-40 yards apart to represent the shores (length of river will depend on size of group). In between the two poles represent the "raging river." Supply a large pile of tools they can choose from (at least enough for one per person) that they will label and use to get the group across the river. Have 2-3 participants be the "alligators" or "piranhas" in the river. Hand the group on the shore 2-3 haltered horses to get across the river.

Briefing:
    This activity is to be a visual for how our own "stuff" can greatly affect our work with our clients if we are aware at all times. You will want to get the group to label all the assets/tools provided as some strength they bring to their profession as an EAP therapist or EAP horse professional.

    Identify the horses as their "clients" throughout the activity when referring to the horses. You can write the label of client on the horse for added visual. Instruct the alligators of their duties while the group is labeling their tools.

GROUP ACTIVITY

Objective:
    To get all of the group and horses across the river using the tools provided.

Rules:
1. No group member can directly touch the "river's water" with any body part or they lose that body part (ie. If they are stepping on a pole and their foot slides off, they lose that foot and must continue without that limb).
2. Must be touching a tool at all time or the tool is at risk of being snatched up by the alligators
3. Must get all group members and all horses across the river
4. Horses are only ones in the group that can walk in the "river's water".
5. Cannot ride the horses
6. Cannot move the shores
7. Alligators cannot go onto the shores
8. Alligators can only get tools that are not in contact with a group member's body part

Instructor's Notes:
1. What did they label as tools? What tools ended up being used? Which ones were left behind? Which ones were snatched by alligators?
2. How did they treat the horses (clients) throughout activity?
3. How creative are they? Did that change when they got frustrated and/or stressed?
4. What themes and patterns are present in their behavior? Any exceptions to behaviors or responses?
5. How did the horses respond?
6. Did they work independently or as a group?
7. What role did the alligators play? Who might those alligators be for the group?
8. What did they do when it got really tense and/ or chaotic?

Debriefing:
1. What was going on for them during that activity?
2. How did the challenges affect their approach to getting the horses (clients) across?
3. What approach did they take to handling alligators in the activity?
4. What might the alligators represent to you?
5. What role did everyone play in the activity and/or in the group?
6. How was this situation similar to their work with their clients?
7. As an EAP professional, what personal applications do they see in this experience?

EXTENDED APPENDAGES
(Kersten and Thomas, 2004)

Type: Group or family (2+ people)

Purpose: Mainly an assessment activity regarding roles, communication, and teamwork

Set-up: It is preferable to have more than one horse in the arena, but one horse is fine as well. Have a halter, lead rope, blanket, and saddle available.

Rules: (3 person family) Have the family line up side by side. Ask them to get connected in some way. – link arms/hold hands/hold clothing. Allow them opportunities to let "connected" look however they choose. Explain to the family that they are like one big body. The person standing in the middle will be the "brains of this operation". The brain is the only one who can think, talk, and give directions. The outside people are the hands (left hand and right hand). As hands, they cannot think, talk, or do anything at all unless the brain directs them (they must remain connected to their brain). The right hand can only use his right hand; the left hand can only use her left hand. All the arms in the middle cannot be used at all (even let the brain know if we see him/her pointing, we will confront her on that, or if the brain has an itch, he/she will have to direct one of her "appendages" to itch it (you can interject humor in your sessions!). In this style, ask the family to catch, halter, and saddle a horse. Let the brain know that directions to the hands need to be specific, and hands need to wait for these specific directions. (e.g. the brain cannot just say, "Halter the horse." The hands do not have brains, so each specific step needs to be described).

Note: You can have a offer the book available on how to saddle if you choose as a recourse. You may or may not make reference to it. This provides opportunities to observe use of resources and awareness of things around them.

Debriefing:
- Look at the non-verbal communication of each person and the horses.
- What happened in the process?
- How did the brain/hands feel in their roles?
- Was their communication from the hands?

FAMILY ACTIVITY

- Was one hand used more than the other?
- Did they work together?
- When did things go the roughest/smoothest?
- Which horse did they choose and why?
- How did the horse respond?
- Tell about the process and about their connections.
- What worked/didn't work?

Variations: Two person format - two people linked, right person directs other's left hand, left person directs other's right hand.

Four person format- Two brains in the middle-right brain directs left hand, left brain directs right hand.

Telephone appendages- One brain, two appendages, the "brain stem"- the rest of the people lined up behind the brain. The person at the end of the "stem" has the book on how to saddle, and is the one who gives the directions. He/she tells the person in front of him/her, who tells the person front of them, who tells the next person, (and so forth), who tells the "brain", who tells the "hands". Issues about bureaucracy and middle management tend to surface in this one! And, I am sure you will come up with many more!

INDIVIDUAL ACTIVITY

VARIATION OF MY WORLD
Musik & Baptis (2002, January/February)

Type: Individual or group therapy

Purpose: Help clients to discover ways and reasons to reach out for support

Materials: 3-5 buckets, 3x5 note cards, and 3 horses

Set-up:
1. This exercise is performed in a round pen with a large circle of feed buckets (3-5) with grain representing good and healthy things in the patient's life that she hold dear i.e., family, friends, dancing, a walk on the beach, etc. Have the patient label each bucket using a 3x5 card.

2. Three horses are used to represent the patient's issues that can rob them of the good and healthy aspects in their life and can be labeled with unhealthy components or specific behaviors using a dry-erase marker on the horse's neck or 3x5 cards attached to each halter i.e., fear, worthlessness, loneliness, addictions, hopelessness, distance from God, weight gain, etc.

3. Depending on if the session is individual or group, another option is to add a support team of two or three persons and have the patient label each member of the team i.e., treatment team, family, God, school, dancing, art, church, etc..

4. Have client build a representation of their "world". Once built they ust stand within that.

Rules: The patient is to keep the horses from robbing her of the things and people she hold dear. Determine the rules in advance and discuss them with participants before the exercise begins.

1. Participants are not to physically touch the horse with body, rocks, etc.
2. This may be a verbal or non-verbal exercise.
3. Goal is to keep horses from eating food
4. Patient must stay within the designated "world" and cannot leave their "world" (represents his/her life).
5. Facilitators may choose whether or not to have support team of two or three persons physically connected (hold hands or link arms).
6. Support team is not allowed to move or help in way until directed by the patient.
7. Patient may utilize only what is inside the round pen.

INDIVIDUAL ACTIVITY

8. Nothing can be removed from the round pen.

Debriefing:

- What took place? Make note of what horse ate or went after what bucket using metaphor's.
- Does he/she spend a lot of time trying to accomplish the goal alone?
- Does the patient quit or give up easily?
- Is he/she frustrated?
- Does he/she ask for help?
- What was the horse's responses to this activity?
- Does the patient use the resources available to accomplish her goal?
- What was the role of the support system? When were the most/least helpful?
- What life applications does this activity hold?

EAP Certification Information

EAGALA has a comprehensive training and certification program in the EAGALA Model of Equine Assisted Psychotherapy and Equine Assisted Learning.

The program involves taking the 3-day Fundamentals of EAGALA Model Practice Part 1 training, the 3-day Fundamentals Part 2 training, and submission of a Professional Development Portfolio. More information on this can be found at www.eagala.org , and dates and locations can be found on the Events page.

Completion of the requirements leads to the designation of "**EAGALA Certified**." Additional training and requirements, including participation in the mentoring program, can be continued to obtain the designation of "**EAGALA Advanced Certified**."
The EAGALA certification requires a renewal every two years which involves continuing education for ongoing learning and development in the model and discipline (EAGALA, 2006).

For the most current certification requirements and level structure visit EAGALA's website at www.eagala.org . Trainings and workshops are taking place worldwide continually, so check EAGALA's calendar for the location nearest you.

EAGALA CODE OF ETHICS

This code serves as a standard of ethics and professionalism for all associates of the Equine Assisted Growth and Learning Association and for the field of Equine Assisted Psychotherapy and Learning. The code delineates basic philosophies to guide professional practitioners in the conduct of business and practice. High standards of ethics and professionalism are established to instill confidence in clients, professionals, and their communities. The ethics code is based on the fundamental values of overall safety and well-being of clients, foremost above all other considerations.

Ethical decisions and conduct should be consistent in the letter and spirit of the code. Failure to act in accordance with the code may result in loss of association or certification with EAGALA. It is our quest to build the emerging field of Equine Assisted Psychotherapy and Learning as a valid, professional, safe, and respected instrument for growth and learning. It is, therefore, required that all practitioners maintain the utmost standards of ethics, professionalism, and integrity.

1. The EAGALA associate will provide the highest quality of service and care in supporting and assisting clients in personal growth and learning.

2. The EAGALA associate will respect and honor the value and dignity of all and protect the safety, welfare, and best interest of the client.

3. The EAGALA associate will always consider physical and emotional safety concerns. This includes safety utilizing horses and the maintenance of a safe facility. Therapeutic approaches are to be implemented in a respectful manner, maintaining the privacy and rights of confidentiality of all clients, and never abusing power through sexual or inappropriate relationships with clients.

4. The EAGALA associate will continually evaluate the progress of clients and will promptly refer them to other professional services if and when this is in the best interest of the client.

5. The EAGALA associate will treat other associates and professionals courteously and respect their views, ideas, and opinions.

6. The EAGALA associate will share information, experiences, and ideas that will benefit, strengthen, and improve the effectiveness of Equine Assisted Psychotherapy.

7. The EAGALA associate will regularly evaluate his/her own professional strengths and limitations and will seek to improve self and profession through ongoing education and training.

8. The EAGALA associate will not misrepresent by claiming or implying professional qualifications, education, experience, or affiliations not possessed by the associate.

9. The EAGALA associate will follow all state/country laws and guidelines pertaining to the scope of his/her practice and limitations of business.

10. The EAGALA associate will not participate in, condone or be associated with dishonesty, fraud, deceit, illegal activities, or misrepresentation.

11. The EAGALA associate will not engage in personal conduct which adversely affects the quality of professional services rendered or cause harm to the reputation of the profession.

12. The EAGALA associate will maintain the highest standards of professional integrity.

© EAGALA, 2006

Bibliography

Aguilera, D. & Messick, J. (1982) Crisis intervention: Theory and methodology (4th ed.). St. Louis: C. V. Mosby.

Ainslie, T. & Ledbetter, B. (1980). The Body Language of Horses. New York: William Morrow and Company, Inc.

Akiyama, A., Holtzman, J., & Britz, W. (1986). Pet ownership and health status during bereavement. Omega, 17, 187-193.

American Counseling Association. (1993). ACA proposed standards of practice and ethical standards. *Guidepost*, 36(4), 15-22.

Anderson, C. (2011, October). The finer points of pressure. Horse and Rider, 28-29.

Anderson, M. (2007, November). Feel your horse's footsteps. Perfect Horse, 12, 18-21.

Anderson, W., Reid, C., & Jennings, G. (1992). Pet ownership and risk factors for cardiovascular disease. Medical Journal of Australia, 157, 298-301.

Angell, J. (1994). The wilderness solo: An empowering growth experience for women. In E. Cole, E. Erdman, & E. D. Rothblum (Eds.), Wilderness therapy for women: The power of adventure (pp. 85 - 100). New York: Haworth Press.

Austin, D. R. (1998). The health protection/health promotion model. Therapeutic Recreation Journal, 109 - 117.

Barker, S., & Dawson, K. (1998). The effects of animal-assisted therapy on anxiety ratings of hospitalized psychiatric patients. Psychiatric Service, 49, 797-801.

Beck, A., Seraydarian, L., & Hunter, G. (1986). The use of animals in the rehabilitation of psychiatric inpatients. Psychological Reports, 58, 63-66.

Beisser, A. R. (1970). The paradoxical theory of change. In J. Fagan & I.L. Shepherd (Eds.), *Gestalt therapy now* (pp. 77-80). New York: Harper & Row (Colophon).

Bennet, B., Bryant, B., VandenBos, G., & Greenwood, A. (1990). Professional liability and risk management. Washington, DC: American Psychological Association.

Benningfield, A.B. (1994). "The impaired therapist." In G.W. Brock (Ed.), American Association for Marriage and Family Therapy ethics casebook (pp. 131-139). Washington DC: American Association for Marriage and Family Therapy.

Berger, K. (2012). The developing person through childhood (6th ed.). New York: Worth Publishers

Boyce, S. & Robertson, D. (2008, Fall). Caution: EAP in progress. EAGALA in Practice, 30-31.

Brabender, V. & Fallon, A. (2009). Group development in practice. American Psychological Association: Washington, D.C.

Bradshaw, J. (1996). Bradshaw on the family: a new way of creating solid self-esteem (revised edition). Deerfield Beach, FL: Health Communications, Inc.

Brammer, L. (1985). The helping relationship: Process and skills (3rd ed.). Upper Saddle River, NJ: Prentice Hall.

Budman, S. H., & Gurman, A. S. (1983). The practice of brief therapy. In Professional Psychology: Research and Practice, 14, no. 3 (pp. 277-292).

Burke, S. (1992). In the presence of animals: Health professionals no longer scoff at the therapeutic effects of pets. U.S. News and World Report, February 24.

Carkhuff, R. & Berenson, B. (1977). Beyond counseling and therapy (2nd ed.). New York: Holt, Rinehart & Winston.

Christie, S. (1997). Seizure-alert dog is girl's lifeline. Dog Fancy, June.

Cherry, K. (2013). What is emotional intelligence? Definitions, history, and measures of emotional intelligence. About.com Psychology. Retrieved on May, 7, 2013 from http://psychology.about.com/od/personalitydevelopment/a/emotionalintell.htm.

Clapp, C. L., & Rudolph, S. M. (1993). Building family teams: An adventure-based approach to enrichment and intervention. In M. A. Gass (Ed.), Adventure therapy: Therapeutic application of adventure programming (pp. 111 - 121). Dubuque, IA: Kendall/Hunt Publishing.

Clay, R. A. (1997). Research reveals the health benefits of pet ownership. APA Monitor, August, 14-15.

Cole, E., Erdman, E., & Rothblum, E (Eds.). (1994). Wilderness therapy for women: the power of adventure. New York: Harrington Park Press.

Cole, K., & Gawlinski, A. (1995). Animal assisted therapy in the intensive care unit. Research Utilisation, 30(3), 529-536.

Connett, M. E. (2008, Spring). Humans step aside: Horses at work. In EAGALA in Practice, pp. 24-26.

Corey, G. (1995). Theory and Practice of Group Counseling. Pacific Grove, CA: Brooks/Cole Publishing Company.

Corey, G., 2009. Theory and Practice of Counseling and Psychotherapy (8th ed.). Pacific Grove, CA: Brooks/Cole Publishing Co.

Corey, G., 1996. Theory and Practice of Counseling and Psychotherapy (5th ed.). Pacific Grove, CA: Brooks/Cole Publishing Co.

Corey, G., Corey, M., Callanan, P. (2011) Issues and Ethics in the Helping Professions (8th ed.). Belmont, CA: Brooks/Cole, CENGAGE Learning.

Corey, G., Corey, M., Callanan, P. (1998) Issues and Ethics in the Helping Professions (5th ed.). Pacific Grove, CA: Brooks/Cole Publishing Co.

Crooks, R. & Stein, J. (1991) Psychology: Science, Behavior & Life. Fort Worth, TX: Holt, Rinehart, & Winston, Inc.

Davis, J. (1988). Animal-facilitated therapy in stress meditation. Holistic Nursing Practice, 2, 75-83.

Davis-Berman, J. & Berman, D. (1994). Wilderness therapy: foundations, theory and research. Dubuque, IA: Kendall/Hunt Publishing.

Davison, G. & Neale, J. (1998). Abnormal Psychology: 7th Edition. New York: John Wiley & Sons, Inc.

de Becker, G. (2002). Fear less: Real truth about risk, safety, and security in a time of terrorism. Little, Brown and Co.

de Shazer, S. (1988). Clues: Investigating solutions in brief therapy. New York: W. W. Norton and Company.

de Shazer, S. (1991). Forward. In Y. M. Dolan, Clues: Investigating solutions in brief therapy, x. New York: W. W. Norton and Company.

Deutsch, C. (1984). Self-reported sources of stress among psychotherapists. <u>Professional Psychology: Research and Practice</u>, 15 (6), 833-845.

Dyk, P., Cheung, R., Pohl, L., Noriega, C., and Lindgreen, J. (2013). <u>The effectiveness of equine guided leadership education to develop emotional intelligence in expert nurses: A pilot research study</u>. Lexington, KY: University of Kentucky Center for Leadership Development.

EAGALA. (2012). <u>Fundamentals of EAGALA Model Practice: Untraining Manual (7th Ed.).</u> Santaquin, UT: EAGALA.

EAGALA. (2010). Standards of each team member in EAGALA Model practice. In <u>EAGALA's Certification Program</u> (Equine Specialist Professional). Retrieved from http://eagala.org/sites/default/files/attachments/EAGALA%20Certification%20Program.pdf

EAGALA. (2006). <u>Fundamentals of EAGALA Model Practice: Untraining Manual (5th Ed.).</u> Santaquin, UT: EAGALA.

Ellis, A. (1988). How to stubbornly refuse to make yourself miserable about anything – Yes, anything! Secaucus, NJ: Lyle Stuart.

Ellis, A. (2001<u>). Overcoming destructive beliefs, feelings, and behaviors</u>. New York: Prometheus Books.

Ellis, A. (2002<u>). Overcoming resistance: A rational emotive therapy integrated approach</u> (2nd Ed.). New York: Springer.

Ellis, A. (1992). Brief therapy: The rational-emotive method. In S.H. Dudman, M.F. Hoyt, & S. Friedman (Eds.), <u>The first session in brief therapy</u> (pp. 26-58). New York: Guilford Press.

Ellis, A., & Dryden, W. (1987). <u>The practice of rational-emotive therapy</u>. New York: Springer.

Egan, G. (1990). <u>The skilled helper</u> (4th Ed.). Pacific Grove, CA: Brooks/Cole.

Erikson, E. (1950). <u>Childhood and Society</u>. New York: Norton.

Feldman, R. (2008). <u>Development across the lifespan</u> (5th Ed.). Upper Saddle River, NJ: Pearson Prentice Hall.

Fisch, R., Weakland, J., and Segal, L. (1982). The tactics of change: Doing therapy briefly. San Francisco: Jossey-Bass.

Fraser, C. (1989, June). Sometimes the best therapy has four legs. RN.

Francis, G., Turner, J., & Johnson, S. (1985). Domestic animal visitation as therapy with adult home residents. International Journal of Nursing Studies, 22 (3), 201-206.

Friedman, E., Katcher, A., Eaton, M., and Berger, B. (1984) Pet ownership and psychological states. In Anderson, R., Hart, B., and Hart, L. (Eds.) The pet connection – Its influence on our health and quality of life (pp. 301-308). Minneapolis: University of Minnesota Press.

Gass, M. A. (1993a). The evolution of processing adventure therapy experiences. In Gass, M. A. (Ed.). Adventure therapy: Therapeutic applications of adventure programming. (pp. 219 - 229). Dubuque, IA: Kendall/Hunt Publishing.

Gass, M. A. (1993b). The theoretical foundations for adventure family therapy. In Gass, M. A. (Ed.). Adventure therapy: Therapeutic applications of adventure programming. (pp. 123 - 137). Dubuque, IA: Kendall/Hunt Publishing.

Gass, M. A. (1993c). Enhancing metaphor development in adventure therapy programs. In Gass, M. A. (Ed.). Adventure therapy: Therapeutic applications of adventure programming. (pp. 245-258). Dubuque, IA: Kendall/Hunt Publishing.

Gelder, B. (2006). Towards the neurobiology of emotional body language. Nature Reviews Neuroscience, 7, 242-249. doi: 10:1038/nrn1872.

Gisch, R., Weakland, J. H., & Segal, L. (1982). The tactics of change: Doing therapy briefly, ix. San Francisco: Jossey-Bass.

Glasser, W. (1985). Control theory: A new explanation of how we control our lives. New York: Harper & Row (Perennial Paperback).

Glasser, W. (1986c). The control theory –reality therapy workbook. Canoga Park, CA: Institue for Control Theory, Reality Therapy, and Quality Management.

Glasser, W. (1989). Control theory in the practice of reality therapy. In N. Glasser (Ed.), Control theory in the practice of reality therapy: Case studies (pp. 1-15). New York: Harper & Row.

Glasser, W. (1992). Reality therapy. New York State Journal for Counseling and Development, 7(1), 5-13.

Goldmeier, J. (1986). Pets or people: Another research note. The Gerontologist, 26(2), 203-206.

Green, M. (1989). Theories of Human Development: A Comparative Approach. Prentice-Hall, Inc.: New Jersey.

Haley, J. (1978). Problem-solving therapy: New strategies for effective family therapy. San Francisco: Jossey-Bass.

Ham, S., Lawrence, K., & Tucker, C. (1998). Teachers don't always have two legs. Paradigm, 2 (3), 4 - 21.

Hamilton, C. (2012, September). On Horses and Autism. America's Horse, pp. 34-36.

Hargrave, J. (1994). Let me see your body talk. Kendall/Hunt Publishing Company.

Hattie, J., Marsh, H. W., Neill, J. T., & Richards, G. E. (1997). Adventure education and outward bound: Out-of-class experiences that make a lasting difference. Review of Educational Research, 67, 43 - 87.

Headey, B., Grabka, M., Kelley, J., Reddy, P., & Tseng, Y. (2002). Pet ownership is good for your health and saves public expenditure too: Australian and German longitudinal evidence. Australian Social Monitor, 5(4), 93-99.

Heady, S. (2003, May/June). Rambling Thoughts about Ethics. EAGALA News, 9.

Hill, C. (2012). 101 ground breaking exercises for every horse and handler. North Adams, MA: Storey Publishing.

Hopkins, D. & Putnam, R. (1993). Personal growth through adventure. London: David Fulton Publishers.

Houck, J., Jung, S., McKissick, D., Hamilton, J., & Lytle, M. (2008, Fall). How does eap work with young children: Can it have a lasting therapeutic effect? EAGALA in Practice, 32-35.

Howe-Murphy, R., & Murphy, J. F. (1987). An exploration of the new age consciousness paradigm in therapeutic recreation. In C. Sylvester, J. L. Hemingway, R., Howe-Murphy, K., Mobily, & P. A. Shank (Eds.). Philosophy of therapeutic recreation: Ideas and issues. Alexandria, VA: National Recreation and Park

Hughes, J. (1993). The effects of adventure-based counseling and levels of sensation on the self-efficacy of chemically dependent males. Doctoral dissertation: Mississippi State University.

Human, L. (2006). Adventure-based experiences during professional training in psychology. South African Journal of Psychology, 36(1), 215-231. 54/07-a of dissertation Abstracts International Abrstract from: DIALOG(R) File 35: Dissertation Abstracts Online, (University Microfilms order # AA094-00484).

Hunter, B., Luna, J., Maglio, D., & Mandrell, R. (2010, Fall). From an ethical perspective, why would EAGALA require a mental health professional to be present in equine assisted learning when it is not about therapy? EAGALA in Practice, 14.

Irwin, C. (Feb. 2000). "Horseplay for Human Potential" In G. Kersten & L. Thomas (Eds.), EAGALA News. Santaquin, UT: EAGALA.

Irwin, C. & Weber, B. (2001). Horses don't lie: What horses teach us about our natural capacity for awareness. Marlow and Company: New York.

James, R. & Gililland, B. (2005). Crisis intervention strategies (5th ed.). New York: Brooks/Cole.

Janosik, E. (1984). Crisis counseling: A contemporary approach. Monterey, CA: Wadsworth Health Sciences Division.

Jensen, A., DeHoff, D., Cordero, F., Haveruk, S., & Mandrell, R. (2008, Spring). The muddiest boots: Finding the right equine specialist. EAGALA in Practice, 20-23.

Kanamori, M., Suzuki, M., Yamamoto, K., Kanda, M., Matsui, Y., Kojima, El, Fukawa, H., Sugita, T., & Oshiro, H. (2001). A day care program and evaluation of animal-assisted therapy (AAT) for the elderly with senile dementia. American Journal of Alzheimers Disease and Other Dementias, 16, 234-239.

Kehler, B. (1998). Challenge Courses and Nature-Based Learning. Christian Counseling Today, 6 (4).

Kelly, D. (2010, Fall). Tom Dorrance: A pioneer for EAP. EAGALA in Practice, 21.

Kersten, G. (1999, April). The "t" in Safety. <u>EAGALA News</u>, 3.

Kersten, G. (1999, July). Creativity vs. Safety. <u>EAGALA News</u>, 3.

Kersten, G. (1999, August). Gate Keeping. <u>EAGALA News</u>, 3.

Kersten, G. (1999, October). Safety Sessions. <u>EAGALA News</u>, 2.

Kersten, G. (1999, November). Cold Weather Concerns. <u>EAGALA News</u>, 2.

Kersten, G. (1999, December). Beware of Wrap Artists. <u>EAGALA News</u>, 2.

Kersten, G., (2000, January). Beyond Punished by Rewards. <u>EAGALA News</u>, 2.

Kersten, G. (2000, February). Making Safety Fun-da-Mental. <u>EAGALA News</u>, 2.

Kersten, G. (2000, July/August). Prior Planning Promotes Prevention. <u>EAGALA News</u>, 2 & 4.

Kersten, G. (2000, September). Safe and Secure. <u>EAGALA News</u>, 2.

Kersten, G. (2003, March/April). Scared Safe. <u>EAGALA News</u>, 2.

Kersten, G. (2004). "Key Ingredients of a Safe Equine Specialist" in Kersten, G. & Thomas, L., <u>Equine-Assisted Psychotherapy and Learning UnTraining Manual.</u> EAGALA: Santaquin, UT.

Kersten, G. (2004, Winter) Reality Safe: Critical Thinking May Reduce Critical Injury. <u>EAGALA News</u>, 2-3.

Kersten, G. & Thomas, L. (2004). Equine-Assisted Psychotherapy and Learning UnTraining Manual: Third Edition. EAGALA: Santaquin, UT.

Kersten, G. & Thomas, L. (1999). Equine-Assisted Psychotherapy and Learning Training Manual, Level 1. EAGALA, Inc.: Santaquin, UT.

Klontz, B., Bivens, A., Leinart, D., Klontz, T. (2007). The effectiveness of equine-assisted experiential therapy: Results of an open clinical trial. <u>Society and Animals, 15</u>, 257-267.

Kohn, A. (1999). Punished by Rewards: The trouble with gold stars, incentive plans, A's, praise, and other bribes. Houghton Mufflin: Boston.

Koss, M. P., & Butcher, J. N. (1986). Research on Brief Psychotherapy. In S. L. Garfield & A. E. Bergin (Eds.), <u>Handbook of Psychotherapy and Behavior Change: An Empirical Analysis (3rd Ed.)</u> (p. 642). New York: John Wiley & Sons.

Kottler, J. & Shepard, D. (2011). <u>Introduction to counseling: Voices of the field. (7th ed.).</u> Belmont: CA: Brooks & Cole, Cengage Learning.

Lancia, J. (2008, Spring). Ascent from hell: EAP in the treatment of war veterans. <u>EAGALA in Practice,</u> 12.

Ledlie, J. A. (Gen. Ed.). (1951). <u>Young adult and family camping</u>. New York: Associated Press.

Leong, F. & Tinsley, H. (Ed.). (2008). <u>Encyclopedia of psychology: Personal and emotional counseling, (Vol. 2.</u>). Thousand Oaks, CA: Sage Publications, Inc.

Levitt, L. (1994). What is the therapeutic value of camping for emotionally disturbed girls? In E. Cole, E. Erdman, & E. D. Rothblum (Eds.), <u>Wilderness therapy for women: The power of adventure</u> (pp. 129 - 138). New York: Haworth Press.

Luckner, J. & Nadler, R. (1997). <u>Processing the experience: Strategies to enhance and generalize learning (2nd Ed.).</u> Dubuque, Iowa: Kendall/Hunt Publishing Co.

Luckner, J. L., & Nadler, R. S. (1995). Processing adventure experiences: It's the story that counts. <u>Therapeutic Recreation Journal, 29 (3),</u> 175 - 183.

Lyons, J. (1998). <u>Communicating with cues: Part I.</u> Greenwich, Connecticut: Belvoir Publications, Inc.

Magnelli, R., Magnelli, N., & Howard, V. (2009, Spring). Case studies. <u>EAGALA in Practice,</u> 38.

Mandrell, P. & Mandrell, R. (2004) <u>Champions: EAP group curriculum for at risk adolescent 10-18 years of age</u> (2nd ed.). Lubbock, TX: Refuge Services, Inc.

Mann, D. (1998). <u>Measuring Outcomes of Equine-Assisted Psychotherapy with Juvenile Delinquents</u>. Unpublished study. Walsenburg, CO.

Mann, J., & Goldman, R. (1973). A casebook in time-limited psychotherapy (p. x.). Cambridge: Harvard University Press.

McMullough, M. (1981). Animal facilitated therapy: Overview and future direction. California Veterinarian, 36, 13-24.

Mearns, D. & Cooper, M. (2005). Working at relational depth in counselling and psychotherapy. London: Sage.

Miles, J. (1993). Wilderness as a healing place. In M. A. Gass (Ed.), Adventure therapy: Therapeutic application of adventure programming (pp. 43 - 55). Dubuque, IA: Kendall/Hunt Publishing.

Miller, R. (1999). Understanding the Ancient Secrets of the Horse's Mind. Neenah, WI: The Russell Murdink Co., Ltd.

Murphy, J. F. (1975). Recreation and services. Dubuque, IA: William C. Brown Company.

Musik, C. & Baptis, L. (2002, January/February). My World. EAGALA News, 7-8.

Myers, D. (2010). *Social Psychology* (10th ed.). New York, New York: McGraw-Hill.

Myers, L. (2009, Spring) Texas rangers. EAGALA in Practice, 18.

Nadler, R. S. (1993). Therapeutic process of change. In M. A. Gass (Ed.), Adventure therapy: Therapeutic application of adventure programming (pp. 57 - 69). Dubuque, IA: Kendall/Hunt Publishing.

Nichols, M. and Schwartz, R. (1998). Family therapy: Concepts and methods (4th Ed.). Boston: Allyn and Bacon.

Oliver, G. J., Hasz, M., & Richburg, M. (1997). Promoting Change through Brief Therapy in Christian Counseling. Wheaton, Illinois: Tyndale House Publishers, Inc.

Oliver, G. J., & Miller, S. (1994). Couple communication. Journal of Psychology and Christianity, 13, 151 - 157.

Pastorino, E. & Doyle-Portillo, S. (2010). What is psychology. Essentials. Belmont, CA: Wadsworth, CENGAGE Learning, 325-328.

Peel, J. & Richards, K. (Dec. 2005). Outdoor Cure. Therapy Today,16(10), 4-8.

Perkins, D. & Salomon, G. (1992). Transfer of learning. <u>International Encyclopedia of Education</u> (2nd Ed.). Oxford, England: Pergamon Press.

Perls, F. (1969a). <u>Gestalt therapy verbatim</u>. Moab, UT: Real People Press.

Piaget, J. (1970). Piaget's theory. In P. Mussen (Ed.), <u>Carmichael's Manual of Child Psychology</u> (Vol. 1). New York: Wiley.

Piaget, J (1971). <u>Genetic epistemology</u>. New York: Norton.

Piaget, J. (1972). Intellectual evolution from adolescence to adulthood. <u>Human Development</u>, 15, 1-12.

Piazza, N. & Baruth, N. (1990). Client record guidelines. <u>Journal of Counseling and Development, 68</u>, 313-316.

Pipher, M. (1996). <u>The shelter of each other: Rebuilding our families</u>. New York: Ballantine Books.

Pommier, J. (1994<u>). Experiential adventure therapy plus family training: outward bound school's efficacy with status offenders.</u> Unpublished doctoral dissertation. Texas: A&M Universery.

Prince, R. (2009, Spring). No fences collaboration. <u>EAGALA in Practice</u>, 32.

Rhoades, J. S. (1972). The problem of individual change in outward bound: An application of change and transfer theory (Doctoral dissertation, University of Massachusetts). <u>Dissertation Abstracts International, 33</u>, 4922A.

Robertson, D. & Boyce, S. (2008, Fall). Caution: EAP in progress. <u>EAGALA in Practice</u>, 30-31.

Rowan, A. & Beck, A. (1994). Editorial: The health benefits of human-animal interactions. <u>Anthrozoos, 72(4)</u>, 85-89.

Saleeby, D. (Ed.). (1992). <u>The strengths perspective in social work practice</u> (p. 171). New York: Longman.

Salovey, P. & Mayer, J. (1990). Emotional intelligence. <u>Imagination, Cognition and Personality, 9</u>, 185-211.

Schultz, P., Remick-Barlow, A., and Robbins, L. (2007). Equine-assisted psychotherapy: A mental health promotion/intervention modality for children who have experienced intra-family violence. <u>Health and Social Care in the Community, 15(3)</u>, 265-271.

Seligman, L. (1990). Selecting effective treatments: A comprehensive systematic guide to treating adult mental disorders. San Francisco, CA: Jossey-Bass.

Shank, J., & Kinney, T. (1987). On the neglect of clinical practice. In C. Sylvester, J. L. Hemingway, R. Howe-Murphy, K. Mobily, & P. A. Shank (Eds.). Philosophy of therapeutic recreation: Ideas and issues. Alexandria, VA: National Recreation & Park.

Shechtman, Z. (2007). Group counseling and psychotherapy with children and adolescents: Theory, research, and practice. Lawrence Erlbaum Associates: Mahwah, NJ.

Shultz, B. (2005). The Effects of equine-assisted psychotherapy on the psychosical functioning of at-risk adolescents ages 12-18. (Counseling thesis, Denver Seminary). Retreived from httm://eagala.org/sites/default/files/attachments/ The%20effects%20of%20Equine-Assisted%20Psychotherapy %20on%20the%20psychosocial%20functioning%20of%20at-risk%20adolescents %20ages%2012-18.pdf.

Siegal, J. (1990). Stressful life events and use of physician services among the elderly: The moderating role of pet ownership. Journal of Personality and Social Psychology, 58(6), 1081-1086.

Sleek, S. (1995, July) Group therapy: Tapping the power of teamwork. APA Monitor, 26(7), 1, 38-39.

Smolowe, A, Butler, S, Murray, M (1999). Adventure in Business. Pearson Custom Publishing.

Sneider, J. (1992). Health muttenance: Pet therapy for elderly, ill. The Business Journal-Milwaukee (September 26).

Sockalingam, S., Li, M., Krishnadev, U., Hanson, K., Balaban, K., Pacione, L., Bhalerao, S. (2008). Use of animal-assisted therapy in the rehabilitation of an assault victim with a concurrent mood disorder. Issues in Mental Health Nursing, 29, 73-84.

Stanley-Hermanns, M., & Miller, J. (2002). Animal-assisted therapy: Domestic animals aren't merely pets. To some they can be healers. American Journal of Nursing, 102(10), 69-76.

Stopha, B. (1994). Women on the ropes: Change through challenge. In E. Cole, E. Erdman, & E. D. Rothblum (Eds.),

Wilderness therapy for women: The power of adventure (pp. 101 - 110). New York: Haworth Press.

Stumbo, N. J., & Peterson, C. A. (1998). The leisure ability model. Therapeutic Recreation Journal, 82 - 96.

Tetreault, A. (2006). Horses that heal: The effectiveness of equine assisted growth and learning on the behavior of students diagnosed with emotional disorder. (Master's Paper, Governors State University). Retreived from httm://eagala.org/sites/default/files/attachments/Horses%20that%20heal:%20The%20effectiveness%20of%20equine%20assisted%20growth%20and%20learning%20on%20the%20behavior%20of%20 students%20diagnosed%20with%20emotional%20disorder.pdf.

Thomas, L. (2012). Countertransference and emotional safety. In EAGALA, Fundamentals of EAGALA Model Practice: Untraining Manual (7th Ed.). Santaquin, UT: EAGALA.

Thomas, L. (Gen. Ed.). (2011). About "'s". In EAGALA in Practice, 4, 3.

Thomas, L. (Gen. Ed.). (2011). Questions and answers. In EAGALA in Practice, 4, 12-13.

Thomas, L. (1999, June). Benefits of EAP. Equine Services News.

Thomas, L & Kersten, G. (2003, January/February). Philosophies on Training, Therapy & Safety. EAGALA News, 2.

Torbert, W. (1972). Learning from experience: Towards consciousness. New York: Columbia University Press.

Torbert, B. (2004). Action inquiry: The secret of timely and transforming leadership. San Francisco: Berrett-Koehler Publishers, Inc.

Trotter, K., Chandler, C., Goodwin-Bond, D., & Casey, J. (2008). A comparative study of the efficacy of group equine assisted counseling with at-risk children and adolescents. Journal of Creativity in Mental Health 3(3), 254-284.

Tucker, M. (1994). Dog Training Made Easy. Howell Book House: New York.

Tyler, J. (1994). Equine psychotherapy: Worth more than just a horse laugh. In E. Cole, E. Erdman, & E. D. Rothblum

(Eds.), <u>Wilderness therapy for women: The power of adventure</u>. New York: Haworth Press.

Voight, A., McCromick, B., & Ewert, A. (2003). Therapeutic outdoor programming: Connections between adventure and therapy. In K. Richards & B. Smith (Eds.), <u>Therapy within adventure</u>. Augsburg: Zeil.

Walsh, K. & Blakeney, B. (2013). Nurse presence enhanced through equus. <u>Journal of Holistic Nursing</u>, Retrieved Jan 28, 2013, <u>www.jhn.sagepub.com/content/early/2013/01/22/0898010112474721</u>.

Walton, R. (1985). Therapeutic camping with inpatient adolescents: a modality for training interpersonal cognitive problem-solving skills. Unpublished doctoral dissertation. St. Louis, MO: Saint Louis University.

Watkins, C. (1983) Transference phenomena in the counseling situation. <u>Personnel and Guidance Journal, 62(4),</u> 206-210.

Watson, W. H. (1997). Soul and system: The integrative possibilities of family therapy. <u>Journal of Psychology and Theology, 25,</u> 123 - 135.

Watzlawick, P., Weakland, J., & Fisch, R. (1974). <u>Change: Principles of problem formation and problem resolution</u>. New York: W. W. Norton and Company.

White, M. (1992). Family therapy training and supervision in world of experience and narrative. In D. Epston and M. White (Eds.), <u>Experience, contradiction, narrative, and imagination</u>. South Australia: Dulwiche Centre Publications.

White, M., & Epston, D. (1990). <u>Narrative means to therapeutic ends</u>. New York: W. W. Norton and Company.

Witman, J. P. (1993). Characteristics of adventure programs valued by adolescents in treatment. <u>Therapeutic Recreation Journal, 27 (1),</u> 44 - 50.

Wolcott, J. (1993). Pet therapy gains credibility in northwest hospitals. <u>Business Journal-Portland, April 19.</u>

Wright, H. N. (1998) Pets in the counseling office. <u>Christian Counseling Today, 6 (4),</u> 28-33.

Wright, D. W., Nelson, B. S., & Georgen, K. E. (1994). Marital problems. P. C. McKenry & S. J. Price (Eds.), Families and change: Coping with stressful events (pp. 40–65). Thousand Oaks, CA: Sage Publications.

Wubbolding, R. E. (2011) Reality therapy: Theories of psychotherapy series. Washington, DC: American Psychological Association.

Young, M. (1992). Counseling methods and techniques: an eclectic approach. Macmillan Publishing Company: New York.

Zimmerman, L. (2010, Fall). Life lessons: Through equine assisted learning. EAGALA in Practice, 32-33.

Zinker, J. (1978). Creative process in gestalt therapy. New York: Random House (Vintage).